T0037463

The Truly Easy Heart-Healthy Cookbook

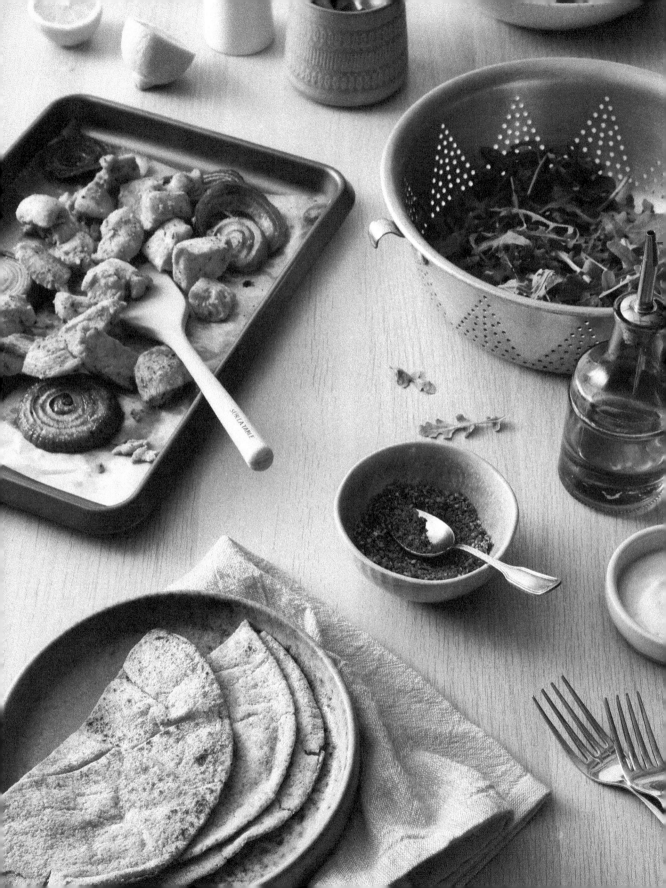

THE TRULY EASY Heart-Healthy

Healthy COOKBOOK

Fuss-Free, Flavorful, Low-Sodium Meals

30-MINUTE, 5-INGREDIENT, and ONE-POT RECIPES

Michelle Routhenstein MS,RD,CDE,CDN

Photography by Laura Flippen

ROCKRIDGE
PRESS

Copyright © 2020 by Rockridge Press, Emeryville, California

No part of this publication may be reproduced, stored in a retrieval system, or transmitted in any form or by any means, electronic, mechanical, photocopying, recording, scanning, or otherwise, except as permitted under Sections 107 or 108 of the 1976 United States Copyright Act, without the prior written permission of the Publisher. Requests to the Publisher for permission should be addressed to the Permissions Department, Rockridge Press, 6005 Shellmound Street, Suite 175, Emeryville, CA 94608.

Limit of Liability/Disclaimer of Warranty: The Publisher and the author make no representations or warranties with respect to the accuracy or completeness of the contents of this work and specifically disclaim all warranties, including without limitation warranties of fitness for a particular purpose. No warranty may be created or extended by sales or promotional materials. The advice and strategies contained herein may not be suitable for every situation. This work is sold with the understanding that the Publisher is not engaged in rendering medical, legal, or other professional advice or services. If professional assistance is required, the services of a competent professional person should be sought. Neither the Publisher nor the author shall be liable for damages arising herefrom. The fact that an individual, organization, or website is referred to in this work as a citation and/or potential source of further information does not mean that the author or the Publisher endorses the information the individual, organization, or website may provide or recommendations they/it may make. Further, readers should be aware that websites listed in this work may have changed or disappeared between when this work was written and when it is read.

For general information on our other products and services or to obtain technical support, please contact our Customer Care Department within the United States at (866) 744-2665, or outside the United States at (510) 253-0500.

Rockridge Press publishes its books in a variety of electronic and print formats. Some content that appears in print may not be available in electronic books, and vice versa.

TRADEMARKS: Rockridge Press and the Rockridge Press logo are trademarks or registered trademarks of Callisto Media Inc. and/or its affiliates, in the United States and other countries, and may not be used without written permission. All other trademarks are the property of their respective owners. Rockridge Press is not associated with any product or vendor mentioned in this book.

Interior and Cover Designer: Darren Samuel
Art Producer: Tom Hood
Editor: Britt Bogan
Production Editor: Nora Milman

Photography © 2020 Laura Flippen

Cover: Zucchini-Chicken Kabobs with Roasted Tomatoes, page 138

ISBN: Print 978-1-64739-315-1 | eBook 978-1-64739-316-8

R0

To my family,
who fills my heart with love
each and every day.

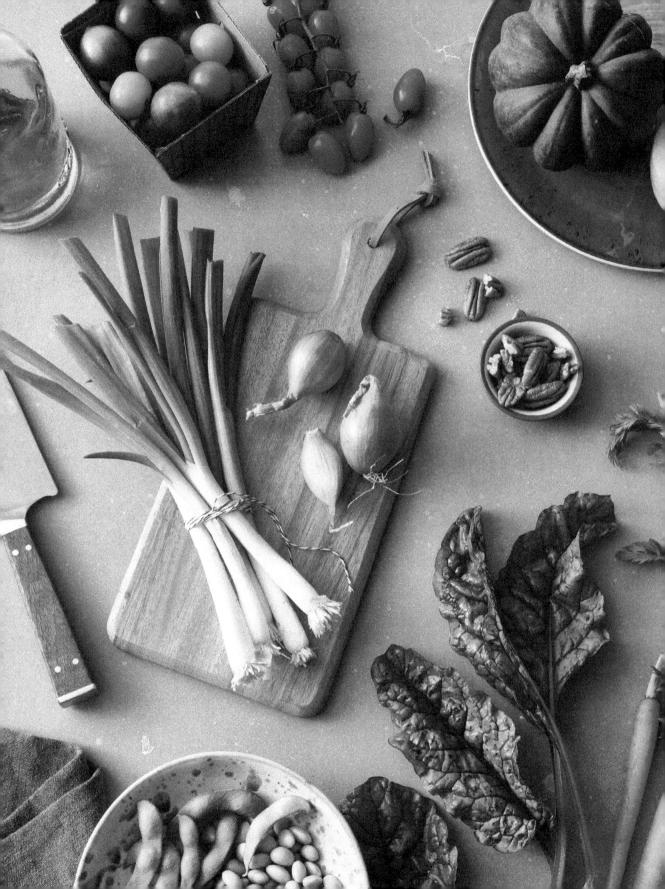

Contents

Introduction

Hi, I'm Michelle, and I am so glad you are here! I am a registered dietitian nutritionist, certified diabetes educator, and preventive cardiology dietitian who specializes in heart-healthy nutrition. I graduated with a master of science in clinical nutrition from New York University (NYU) and completed my dietetic residency at NYU. I have over 10 years' experience counseling individuals on chronic disease prevention and management. I currently see clients in my private practice, Entirely Nourished, in New York City and virtually.

In my practice, I have seen people struggle with the what, where, and how to eat heart-healthy. I understand that a cardiac diet can be overwhelming and confusing. Many of my clients come to me not knowing where to begin. They have heard of many foods to avoid, but they feel unsure of what foods to actually eat. The idea of reducing salt, fat, and meat from one's diet seems intimidating, tasteless, and hard to do.

I have successfully helped thousands of people lower their blood pressure and cholesterol levels and have even had many reduce or completely get off their blood pressure and statin medications through heart-healthy diet changes.

I am here to help you eat heart-healthy in a simple, easily approachable manner that still allows you to enjoy food while protecting your heart. I break down the science of what constitutes a heart-healthy diet and incorporate it into the recipes so you don't have to. A heart-healthy diet should be easy, quick, and flavorful so you can enjoy the food you eat and adapt it into your life forever.

The recipes found in this book adhere to a mixture of researched-backed heart-healthy diets such as the DASH, the Mediterranean, and a vegetarian diet. These diets emphasize macronutrient balance and consumption of vital micronutrients to protect your heart and help with optimal blood flow and blood vessel function.

All the recipes found in this book are easy in a variety of ways: 30 minutes or less, one-pot, and 5-ingredient meals. You can choose the version of easy that best suits you. All of the recipes rely on fresh, healthy, affordable, and easy-to-find ingredients.

Whole Wheat Couscous Tabbouleh with Pomegranate Seeds

PAGE 57

One

EATING HEART-HEALTHY MADE EASY

Welcome to heart-healthy eating! This chapter lays out the nuts and bolts of eating heart-healthy and provides the info and tools to do so easily. It also covers some frequently asked questions; touches on some common heart medications and food interactions; provides a list of fresh, frozen, and pantry essentials; and offers shopping shortcuts and meal-planning tips. You'll learn how to make quick and flavorful heart-healthy food without added salt and fat.

Love Your Heart Through Food

Everyone is at a different stage of their heart-health journey. Some of you may have an official diagnosis, some may be recovering from cardiac surgery, and others might use this as a preventative measure.

Nutrition is the most powerful tactic you can utilize to heal your body and protect your heart. There are certain foods that can negatively contribute to heart disease and clog your arteries, causing restriction of blood flow and narrowing of blood vessels. These foods are high in trans fat, which is primarily found in fried foods and hydrogenated oils; saturated fat, which is primarily found in meats like beef, pork, and lamb; processed meats like hot dogs, salami, and sausages; and high-fat dairy products like cheese, butter, whole milk, and ghee. However, there are many foods that are needed for your body and heart to function properly and improve blood flow and blood vessel health.

Heart-healthy foods include rich sources of antioxidants and polyphenols that protect the heart against harmful stresses (such as quercetin in fennel and anthocyanins in red cabbage and berries), nitric oxide–containing foods that increase blood flow (such as arugula, kale, garlic, sesame seeds, and pumpkin seeds), omega-3–rich foods that fight inflammation (such as salmon and sardines), B vitamin–rich foods that help stabilize plaque formation (such as chickpeas, lean chicken breast, and edamame), fiber-rich foods that help promote proper excretion of excess cholesterol from the body (such as whole grains, fruits, and vegetables), fresh herbs and spices that reduce swelling (such as turmeric and garlic), and magnesium and potassium-rich foods that help maintain a proper heartbeat, heart function, and blood pressure (such as avocados, lentils, and dark chocolate).

I understand that any kind of diet and lifestyle change isn't easy, but I am here to help smooth the way by providing clear instructions and delicious examples.

CARING FOR A LOVED ONE

I can empathize with the gravity of caring for someone with heart disease. Managing that and your own life may feel like a huge task. So, here are five tips for caregivers to make things a bit easier:

Make one meal for everyone. If you make one meal for the whole family, you'll free up a lot of your time and reduce stress. If others really want to add more salt, they can adjust on their own.

Go to the grocery store prepared. Try discussing two to four meals to make for the week. Involving your loved one in the process allows them to feel heard, which can help encourage them to eat the meals. Write out the days of the week, the meals planned for each, and the groceries needed.

Make leftovers your friend. Pick one or two days to meal prep. Double the recipe of a particular dish your loved one enjoys most and freeze it in individual portions so they can easily thaw and warm it up as needed. Consider preassembling smoothie or meal ingredients and sauces to make meal prep even quicker.

Be supportive, even if they eat something they're "not supposed to." You don't want them to hide things from you. Ask if there is a way you can make a healthier version more appealing. You can ask them what flavor profile they are in the mood for, and then you can easily add that flavor element to a snack or meal. By listening to them and their preferences, they feel supported in their journey.

Have a favorite seasoning blend. Make a go-to seasoning blend, so that when you're in a pinch, they can add flavor to their own food by using a dash of the salt-free spice blend.

What Does a Heart-Healthy Diet Look Like?

In this section, we'll address the popular and well-documented heart-healthy diets and the common questions people have about eating heart-healthy.

MEDITERRANEAN, DASH, AND PLANT-BASED DIETS

Although there isn't one best heart-healthy diet, many prominent medical establishments, including the American College of Cardiology, generally agree that plant-based diets such as the Mediterranean, DASH (Dietary Approaches to Stop Hypertension), and vegetarian diets are the heart-healthiest ways to eat. This book's recipes all comply with at least one of these three diets.

Plant-based diets are heart-healthy because they significantly reduce the consumption of many animal products that are high in artery-clogging saturated fat and trimethylamine N-oxide derivatives, such as red meat. Plant-based diets are also cardio-protective because the foods abundantly recommended contain heart-healthy vitamins, minerals, fiber, polyunsaturated fats, and anti-inflammatory antioxidants.

Plant-based diets emphasize plant foods, while de-emphasizing some animal products. A vegetarian diet removes meat and sometimes fish, dairy, and eggs. The Mediterranean and DASH diets are rich in vegetables, fruits, nuts, beans, seeds, whole grains, low-fat or nonfat dairy, and have moderate amounts of fish and poultry. The Mediterranean diet emphasizes red wine consumption and monounsaturated fats (such as olive oil), while the DASH diet emphasizes sodium reduction.

The DASH diet protects the heart by helping lower blood pressure in individuals with high blood pressure, along with reducing bad LDL cholesterol and improving insulin resistance. High blood pressure means too much pressure is placed on the blood vessel walls, leading to stressed, overworked arteries that can scar and be more susceptible to plaque buildup—increasing the risk of blood clots, stroke, and heart disease. This diet emphasizes sodium reduction along with an increase in potassium, magnesium, and calcium for optimal blood vessel health.

The Mediterranean diet mirrors the DASH diet and emphasizes consuming moderate amounts of monounsaturated fat from extra-virgin olive oil, avocados, and certain nuts. In the PREDIMED study, the diet's extra heart-healthy monounsaturated fat reduced the risk of cardiovascular events by about 30 percent compared to a low-fat diet. Replacing saturated fat with monounsaturated fat also significantly decreases LDL and triglyceride levels—if either parameter is elevated, it can increase the risk of a stroke or heart attack.

WHAT ABOUT LOW-CARB DIETS?

Low-carbohydrate diets, specifically the ketogenic and paleo diets, replace carbohydrates with fat and therefore are not optimal heart-healthy diets. The ketogenic diet can restrict carbohydrates to 20 to 50 grams per day, which is dangerously low for optimal brain and heart function. The National Academy of Medicine established a recommended daily intake of at least 130 grams per day for adults to achieve the needed amount of glucose for the brain to function properly. Additionally, these diets can contain up to 70 to 80 percent total calories from fat, with a large quantity of artery-clogging saturated fat. Low-carbohydrate diets can also place you at risk for deficiencies of vitamins and minerals such as potassium, magnesium, folate, biotin, thiamin, selenium, and vitamins A and E.

WHAT IF I HAVE A CROSSOVER CONDITION?

Many individuals dealing with heart disease may also have another condition that can further impact the way they eat. For instance, some may have prediabetes, diabetes, or insulin resistance, and should also focus on carbohydrate type and amount, along with dietary fiber. Others may have varying stages of chronic kidney disease and may have to focus on their individual needs for protein, potassium, phosphorus, and fluid consumption to avoid overtaxing their kidneys. For those managing their weight, I would recommend to particularly home in on hunger and satiety cues before and after meal consumption. Meeting one on one with a registered dietitian can help individuals achieve optimal results by simultaneously addressing an individual's chronic conditions, lifestyle factors, and food preferences.

WHAT IF I AM RECOVERING FROM HEART SURGERY?

Cardiac surgery has been shown to create a cascade of inflammatory responses, which can lead to more complications, such as multiple-organ injury and dysfunction. Adequate and balanced post-surgery nutrition is important for various reasons, including reducing post-operative complications and improving wound healing. Specific, well-researched studies show that protein, vitamins D and C, and selenium are stressed as being integral components of an optimal post-surgery diet. If you don't have an appetite and cannot eat large meals, consume small meals more frequently to obtain all the necessary nutrients to protect your heart and promote functional recovery and healing.

HEART MEDICATIONS AND FOOD INTERACTIONS

If you're taking medication, there are some food-drug interactions to be aware of. Talk to your doctor about any medications you're taking and potential dietary changes.

Statins with Grapefruit or Pomegranate

Grapefruit has a high concentration of furanocoumarins, which are plant-based compounds that block the enzyme needed to break down specific statins (a class of drugs that lower cholesterol levels) and calcium channel blockers (a class of blood pressure medications). Grapefruit may increase blood levels of a statin by 8 to 260 percent and may reduce calcium channel blocker effectiveness by about half. Furanocoumarins are also found in pomegranates and may have the same effect.

Coumadin (Warfarin) and Vitamin K

Oftentimes vitamin K is looked at as a vitamin to avoid if you are taking Coumadin, a blood-thinning medication; I want to debunk this myth. First, vitamin K is needed in blood clotting when a blood vessel is injured, and a deficiency can increase the risk of excess bleeding. A deficiency can also cause an increase in calcium buildup in the heart because vitamin K is needed to efficiently place calcium in the bones.

Coumadin reduces blot clotting by blocking vitamin K-dependent blood-clotting factors. Your blood's ability to clot is closely monitored by testing your clotting time, also known as your international normalized ratio (INR) lab test. The doctor will adjust your Coumadin dosage to keep your INR within a target range. Therefore, vitamin K intake needs to be consistent for the Coumadin dosage to be tightly regulated, and a sudden change is not advised. In addition, consuming high-dose supplements of garlic, turmeric, ginkgo biloba, St. John's wort, vitamin E, and/or omega-3 fatty acids with blood-thinning medications can be dangerous. Taking these supplements together with these medications can thin your blood to extremely dangerous levels and may increase your risk of internal bleeding.

The Heart of the Heart-Healthy Diet

A heart-healthy diet's essence is balance: lean protein, heart-healthy fats, and complex carbohydrates. The goal is to decrease the consumption of artery-clogging foods and add nutrient-rich cardioprotective foods that are plentiful in vitamins, minerals, and antioxidants. Here are a few guiding principles:

Eat lean protein. Lean protein includes legumes, beans, egg whites, omega-3–rich fish, low-fat dairy, and chicken breast. Adding in more nonprocessed, plant-based options is an easy way to actively reduce inflammation. Lean protein also adds a host of cardioprotective vitamins and minerals, such as potassium, magnesium, selenium, and vitamin B$_6$.

Choose unsaturated fat over saturated fat. Prioritizing unsaturated fats over trans and saturated ones helps remove bad cholesterol and increase good cholesterol. Unsaturated fats include avocados, avocado oil, olive oil, nuts, seeds, and omega-3–rich fish. Portions need to be monitored because fat has more calories than protein and carbohydrates, but a small portion is encouraged at each meal.

Pick complex carbs high in dietary fiber. Dietary fiber protects your heart by significantly reducing your total cholesterol and LDL levels. Studies show every additional 7 grams of dietary fiber per day may lower your cardiovascular disease risk by 9 percent. Complex carbohydrates such as vegetables, whole grains, beans, legumes, and fruits contain varying amounts of soluble and insoluble fiber. Soluble fiber traps carbohydrates and bile acids during digestion, and insoluble fiber allows for proper elimination. Both soluble fiber and insoluble fiber work in tandem to reduce blood sugar and lipid levels and keep your arteries clean.

Prioritize antioxidants. Consuming an antioxidant-rich diet also helps reduce inflammation. Inflammation promotes plaque growth that clogs arteries and may cause blood clots, thereby increasing the risk of heart attacks and strokes. Making dishes that are antioxidant-rich and feature vegetables and high-fiber fruits is an easy way to help lower inflammation in your body.

Reduce your salt intake. Low-sodium diets are a mainstream recommendation in heart-healthy diets, and they are backed by significant research. While we need to focus on a low-sodium diet, we also need to emphasize the importance of adding in fresh herbs (such as basil and dill), spices (such as oregano and garlic), and flavorful foods (such as onions and leeks) to make foods enjoyable and tasty. Consuming potassium-rich foods, such as cooked spinach, cooked broccoli, and sweet potatoes, helps eliminate excess sodium in your body, which helps lower blood pressure and improve circulation.

Bake, steam, and roast your way to success. Your meal's preparation can significantly impact your blood pressure and cholesterol management. Swap deep-fried foods for foods that are baked, steamed, roasted, or grilled for a boost in nutrient absorption and optimal blood-vessel health.

Attune to your hunger cues. Maintaining a healthy metabolic rate and body weight by listening to your body's hunger and satiety cues also lessens the stress on your heart. Consuming food within one hour of waking up and timing food consumption based off your hunger signals is imperative to keeping your metabolism revved through the day and as you age. When you are slightly hungry, you should eat, and when you are slightly satisfied, you should stop.

Consuming a heart-healthy diet can be easily implemented by eating more cardio-protective foods and limiting foods that add stress to your heart and circulatory system. See the following charts for a comprehensive list.

Foods to Love, Limit, and Let Go

This table looks at different categories of foods to love, limit, and let go of. The "To Love" category represents a better choice for your heart when eaten in moderation as part of a well-balanced meal. Grains should still be limited to ⅓ to ½ cup per serving and dairy, fish, poultry, and soy to about 4 to 6 ounces per serving, depending on the individual.

FOODS TO LOVE

GRAINS
Whole grains such as oats, quinoa, farro, bulgur, buckwheat, whole wheat couscous, whole wheat pasta, whole barley, and brown rice

DAIRY
Organic nonfat and low-fat yogurt, kefir, milk

FISH
Wild salmon, Arctic char, sardines, bronzini, halibut, rainbow trout, Pacific cod, Atlantic sea bass, and barramundi

POULTRY AND MEATS
Skinless chicken breast, skinless lean turkey breast, lean or very lean ground chicken or turkey

SOY
Organic tofu, tempeh, edamame, cooked soybeans, and soymilk

LEGUMES
Sprouted and boiled beans, canned beans (no salt added, low-sodium, or rinsed, all BPA-free), or Tetra Pak low-sodium beans

NUTS AND SEEDS
Raw and unsalted nuts and seeds (such as walnuts, almonds, pistachios, chia seeds, flaxseed, and pumpkin seeds), nut butters with only the nut on the ingredient list

VEGETABLES
All fresh and frozen vegetables (with no added salt)

FRUITS
All fresh or frozen fruit (with no added sugar)

OILS
Olive oil, avocado oil

BEVERAGES
Water and teas, specifically green tea, black tea, oolong tea, and hibiscus tea

FOODS TO LIMIT

Whole wheat bread, whole wheat sourdough

Part-skim mozzarella cheese, ricotta cheese, and feta cheese in water

Mackerel, tuna, red snapper, and shellfish

Skinless chicken thighs, skinless chicken drumstick

Miso

N/A

Nut and seed flours

Pureed vegetables and soups (as they lose intact fiber when pureed)

No-sugar-added dried fruit

Sesame oil

Coffee and red wine

FOODS TO LET GO

Refined carbohydrates such as high-sugar cereals, white rice, white flour pasta, and white breads

Hard cheeses, especially processed cheese such as Velveeta, full-fat dairy, coconut yogurt, and yogurt with added sugar

Tilapia, flounder, swordfish, tilefish, shark, herring in tartar sauce, and anchovies

Fried chicken; deli and processed meats such as bacon and sausage; and red meat, especially fatty cuts of meat such as heavily marbled meats, rib eye steak, strip steak, and skirt steak

Processed soy such as textured soy protein, soy protein isolate, soy sauce, tamari sauce, and soybean oil

High-sodium canned beans and refried baked beans

Processed nut butters with hydrogenated oils or palm oil, prepackaged salted and roasted seeds or nuts

French fries, tempura-battered vegetables, creamed or high-salt canned or frozen vegetables

Sugar-added dried fruit, jams, and juices

Vegetable shortening, hydrogenated oils, palm oil, coconut oil, margarine, ghee, and butter

Soda, diet soda, energy drinks, and juices

Shopping Shortcuts and Planning Pro Tips

The first step to cooking heart-healthy is to shop smart and plan ahead. You may no longer be able to rely on some of the shortcuts you took before, such as using high-sodium bottled sauces or ordering takeout if you didn't plan dinner. Here are some ways to make heart-healthy shopping and meal planning easier.

Plan out the week ahead and have a grocery list. Decide what recipes you'll make for the week and write a grocery list with the items you need. Consider choosing recipes with ingredients that overlap and buying those items in bulk.

Buy frozen or pre-cut vegetables. To lessen prep time and avoid the extra salt in canned vegetables, buy frozen vegetables or bagged, pre-chopped vegetables instead. Many stores also have vegetables cut into strips, which can make an easy slaw. A report prepared by the Environmental Quality and Food Safety Research Unit at the University of Chester showed that some vegetables, particularly frozen broccoli, carrots, and Brussels sprouts, contained more vitamin C, lutein, and beta-carotene than fresh!

Have a go-to spice blend. Make a seasoning blend of spices you enjoy and have it on hand to quickly season lean protein without the added sodium. I really like savory, so a Mediterranean blend of paprika, cumin, turmeric, and black pepper is a staple in my home. With your favorite spice blend, you can make simple and easy meals by shaking the blend over a protein, vegetables, and a whole grain carbohydrate, and then cooking them in a heart-healthy way.

Cook in bulk. Double batch and freeze herbs, sauces, or parts of a meal so you can eliminate a step in the cooking process when you are in a pinch for time. For example, cut up a whole bunch of basil and divide it into 1-teaspoon increments in ice cube trays; add water and freeze for easy use. Next time you need it to spice up a dish or make a quick pesto sauce, easily defrost it in the actual pan or overnight in the refrigerator. You can also prep and pre-pack smoothie ingredients to make a quick breakfast smoothie in the morning.

Keep pantry staples on hand. Keep a stock of frozen essentials and pantry staple items such as low-sodium, Tetra Pak canned beans and frozen vegetables. Stocking these staples means you'll have all the ingredients for an easy meal if you don't have time to cook or find that you've forgotten an ingredient that you can easily replace with something else.

Repurpose leftovers. If you're having chicken, fish, tofu, or a bean dish for dinner you can take the leftovers and shred them, or just add them to the top of a salad for another meal. If you have leftover salad or vegetables, throw them in a pot with your favorite heart-healthy protein for an easy balanced meal.

READING NUTRITION LABELS

Reading a product's nutritional label is as important as reading its ingredients. A nutritional label is a chart on the back of most packaged foods that details the ingredients and nutritional content of the item. Items to pay close attention to include saturated and trans fats, sodium, carbohydrates, dietary fiber, and added sugar. Saturated fats should be limited to 2 grams or less per serving due to its artery-clogging effect. Avoid trans fats completely because they accelerate atherosclerosis; aim for 0 grams. Check the ingredients list for "hydrogenated oils"; if those are in the list, leave it on the shelf. Limit sodium to 150 milligrams per snack serving and 300 milligrams per meal serving because of its negative arterial effects.

Carbohydrates are necessary because they contribute dietary fiber and essential vitamins and nutrients; however, consume them in moderation to avoid weight gain and minimize plaque formation. First look at the total carbohydrates, it should be between or less than 15 to 20 grams of carbohydrates per serving in a snack or between or less than 30 to 45 grams of carbohydrates in a meal, after accounting for dietary fiber. To account for the dietary fiber, subtract the total grams of carbohydrates from the total grams of fiber. For instance, a slice of bread may contain 20 grams of carbohydrates and 5 grams of dietary fiber; the total net carbohydrates would be 15 grams. Aim for dietary fiber to be at least 4 grams in a whole grain food, such as high-fiber cereals or whole wheat breads.

Added sugars include any sugars that are added to your food during the processing or packaging process, and should be limited as much as possible. The American Heart Association recommends the maximum amount of sugar consumption be about 6 teaspoons (25 grams) per day for women and about 9 teaspoons (37.5 grams) per day for men.

Find the Easiest Cooking Method for You

This book is easy in three different ways, so you can pick the one that best suits you: 5 ingredients (excluding oil, salt, water, and pepper), meaning less prep; 30-minute meals (or less), meaning a quick cook time; and one-pot, meaning less cleanup. Everyone's idea of easy is different and what may be easy one day may not be easy the next. For instance, on weeknights, you may choose a 30-minute meal, and on weekends, you might prefer a one-pot meal, even if it needs to cook for a little bit longer.

EFFORTLESS WAYS TO BOOST FLAVOR WITHOUT ADDED SALT AND FAT

One of the biggest complaints about heart-healthy foods is that they are flavorless and bland. I have endeavored to ensure that all the recipes are tasty and full of flavor without adding unhealthy fats or salt. One of the ways I boost flavor in some of the recipes is by combining aromatics such as garlic, shallots, ginger, and leeks with fresh herbs in a sauce, such as a Cilantro-Mint Sauce (page 163) or a pesto sauce, to top a dish. Flavor is also created by blending and marrying spices to make, for instance, a barbeque flavor or chile-lime flavor, without the added salt. Cooking methods such as broiling, roasting, and pan-searing enable the natural sugars in the vegetables to add a robust flavor. Many times the dish does not need much oil, but rather needs a liquid to cook in; citrus juices, water, broth, or a nut or seed base are used to cut the fat and make a dish delicious. This also allows you to easily mix and match different sauces, proteins, vegetables, and flavors to complement your or your loved one's mood and taste buds. Just be mindful the cooking times may vary depending on the swap.

A Simple Heart-Healthy Kitchen

This section guides you through the fresh and frozen staples and basic kitchen tools you will need to cook heart-healthy meals.

FRESH AND FROZEN ESSENTIALS

These vegetables, proteins, and fats are the building blocks to have on hand to have a heart-healthy kitchen at the ready. This book's recipes mix and match these ingredients, so if you have them, you'll be ready to whip something up at any time.

Alliums: Onions, garlic, leeks, shallots, scallions, and chives are all part of the allium family, and they all add tons of flavor to any dish. Onions and garlic both contain S-nitrosoglutathione, which promotes nitric oxide, a blood flow–improving vasodilator. Choose firm and dry onions with intact, shiny skin and no soft spots. Choose tight garlic without any broken skin or damp or soft spots; the firmer the garlic, the more flavorful it will be. Garlic and onions are best stored in a cool, dry, and well-ventilated place. You can also easily substitute garlic and onions for leeks or shallots in most dishes. If you are allergic to alliums, consider swapping in celery root, fennel, or green peppers instead.

Avocados: Avocados are composed of heart-healthy monounsaturated fats, particularly inflammation-reducing oleic acid (the same monounsaturated fat found in olive oil) that has been linked to heart benefits when it replaces saturated fat. Avocados can help create a creamy salad dressing, balance the texture and taste of a dish, or be served as a dip with crudité. If you plan to use the avocado immediately, choose one that is lightly soft (not mushy) when squeezed. Placing it in the refrigerator will help slow down the ripening process for an extra day or two. If you are buying avocados to use later in the week, choose slightly firm avocados and leave them on your countertop to ripen. The darker the color, generally the more ripe it will be; however, some avocado varieties differ in color and this may not always hold true.

Berries: Berries are rich in dietary fiber, vitamin C, manganese, and inflammation-reducing anthocyanins and polyphenols. Berries such as strawberries, blackberries, blueberries, and raspberries are great to have fresh when they are in season, and frozen are just as good year-round. When buying fresh berries, inspect the entire container—especially the bottom half—for any moisture or mold. When shopping frozen, ensure that the ingredients list only includes berries with no added sugar or preservatives.

Citrus: Citrus fruits such as lemons, limes, and tangerines help flavor and add complexity to dishes. Pick a medium to large lemon or lime with thin skin for a sweeter, juicier fruit. Look for fruits that are bright in color without any discoloration or spots. Squeeze the fruit gently with your thumb, and it should give back a little bit. It is best stored in a refrigerator drawer, or you can squeeze a batch into ice cube trays and have it available to you in your freezer for a quick addition to a dish.

Cruciferous vegetables: Cruciferous vegetables belong to the *Brassica* species and include broccoli, cabbage, bok choy, cauliflower, Brussels sprouts, radish, and turnips. Many contain sulforaphane, which helps reduce inflammation and prevents narrowing of the arteries. When purchasing these fresh, make sure they smell fresh and don't have any browning or wet spots. If buying them frozen, ensure the veggies don't have any added salt, fat, flavoring, or cream.

Eggs or 100-percent-liquid egg whites: Eggs are packed with a beautiful heart-healthy profile of B vitamins, selenium, choline, lutein, zeaxanthin, and possibly omega-3 fatty acids (depending on which you purchase). But they do contain some cholesterol. However, most people's actual cholesterol profile with not change from moderate egg consumption. In fact, some studies even show that eggs increase HDL (good cholesterol) and change the bad cholesterol to a large subtype that's good for the heart. The American Heart Association states that consuming one whole egg a day (or seven eggs a week) can be part of a heart-healthy diet. Studies show the best quality eggs are ones that come from pasture-raised, grass-fed chickens with deep yellow-orange yolks. For ease of use, 100-percent-liquid egg whites can be a quick substitute.

Fresh fish: Many fish, such as wild salmon, sardines, Arctic char, and rainbow trout, are particularly rich in anti-inflammatory omega-3 fatty acids. Consuming omega-3 fatty acid–rich fish two to three times a week has been shown to reduce the risk of cardiovascular disease. When shopping for salmon, choose wild versus farm-raised because wild salmon has a healthier ratio of anti-inflammatory omega-3s compared to pro-inflammatory omega-6 fatty acids. Farm-raised salmon may also have higher contaminants, such as carcinogenic dioxins and Polychlorinated Biphenyls (PCBs).

Fresh herbs: Many fresh herbs, such as basil, dill, parsley, and cilantro, have heart-healthy nutrients and antioxidants that nourish your body and your palate. Inspect the leaves and stems for a healthy, blemish-free appearance; they should resemble a living plant. The best way to check for a flavorful herb is to smell it; it should have a very clean and pleasant smell. For best storage, cut about ½ inch off the end of the stems and place them in a water-filled glass in the refrigerator. Alternatively, tightly wrap them in a paper towel and place them in an airtight container. You can also store fresh herbs in the freezer by first dicing them, then adding them to ice cube trays and filling up ¼ of the ice cube tray with water.

Green leafy vegetables: Green leafy vegetables are particularly abundant in heart-healthy nutrients such as magnesium, manganese, potassium, vitamin K, and folate. Some are also particularly high in vasodilating nitric oxide, such as kale, arugula, Swiss chard, and spinach. Check all your greens before you buy them to make sure they aren't limp or wilted. If purchasing them in bags or plastic boxes, the herbs or vegetables should appear dry and shouldn't have excess condensation inside them. If they are pre-washed, extend their shelf life by rolling them in a paper towel and sealing them in an airtight container.

Low-fat plain yogurt: Organic, low-fat (0 to 2 percent) Greek yogurt is an easy protein to add to meals, smoothies, or dips. Whenever possible, choose organic, pasture-raised dairy. Organic, pasture-raised dairy may have more iron and polyunsaturated fat content, particularly omega-3 fatty acids, than conventional dairy.

Tofu: Tofu is a high-quality plant-based protein made from condensed soymilk that is formed into solid white blocks and is rich in manganese, calcium, selenium, and magnesium. It can be used in just about any dish because it takes on the flavor of the dish's ingredients. It also contains heart-healthy isoflavones, a potent antioxidant that reduces inflammation and improves blood vessel health and arterial elasticity. A study in the *American Journal of Clinical Nutrition* showed that regular consumption of one ounce of tofu lowered the risk of heart disease by 10 percent. When picking tofu, choose organic if you are able to. Firm and extra-firm tofu are dense and hold their shape, making them a good choice for a stir-fry, soup, or grilled dish. Soft tofu has a smoother texture that's good for dips or spreads. Silken tofu is very soft and can be used in sauces or as a substitution for eggs, creams, and yogurt.

Unsalted nuts and seeds: Unsalted nuts and seeds are a great addition to salads, soups, and main dishes, and they may improve blood vessel function, while decreasing inflammation and oxidative stress. Keep one to three varieties on hand, as each nut and seed has different heart-healthy qualities, including unsaturated oil, which can become rancid at room temperature. It is best to store them in the refrigerator for up to six months or in the freezer for up to a year.

PANTRY ESSENTIALS

These 10 ingredients are great shelf-stable cupboard items to have handy to easily flavor a meal and make prep quicker when in a pinch for time.

Avocado oil: Avocado oil is rich in oleic acid, a monounsaturated fat that may help reduce blood pressure levels. Avocado oil has a high smoke point, which means that the heart-healthy fat composition won't change during cooking. It doesn't have much of a taste, but it adds heart-healthy benefits and allows for cooking at higher heats. Make sure you purchase 100-percent-pure avocado oil and not a mixture of a variety of oils.

Balsamic vinegar: Balsamic vinegar is a concentrated vinegar made with grape must. It has a sweet, tart taste that complements salads and certain desserts. Balsamic vinegar contains acetic acid, which has probiotic-like benefits that may aid digestion and keep your gut microbiome healthy. To choose the best balsamic vinegar, read the ingredient label. It should just say "grape must and vinegar." If it is made with red wine vinegar, it will be more bitter. The longer it has aged, the more flavorful and complex it is. Store in a cool, dark place.

Canned fish: Wild salmon, sardines, and tuna are easy staples to have on hand, making meals in a pinch with high-quality omega-3 fatty fish. Choose Tetra Pak or BPA-free, no salt added, packed in water varieties to ensure a low-sodium option. While sardines are often ignored, they provide an easy way to get in those highly talked about omega-3 fatty acids, while also being a good source of vitamin B_{12}. Keep canned sardines in water available so you can easily add them to a salad or vegetable dish for a high-quality, lean, nutrient-dense option.

Dark chocolate: Dark chocolate's heart-healthy benefits are derived from its antioxidant-packed cacao content. Dark chocolate with at least 70 to 85 percent of cacao is rich in dietary fiber, iron, magnesium, copper, and manganese. Make sure the first ingredient is cacao beans and avoid alkalized or "Dutched" dark chocolate because that process significantly decreases the chocolate's antioxidants; if the ingredient label says "cocoa processed with alkali," avoid that product. Choose organic and fair trade whenever possible because harvesting cacao beans is an arduous process, and pesticides can easily affect the quality.

Dried spices: Spices are rich in antioxidants and many have cardioprotective anti-inflammatory properties. Dried spices such as black pepper, turmeric, paprika, cumin, garlic, cayenne pepper, and cinnamon make dishes flavorful without the salt. Spices should always have a fragrant flavor. If the aroma is dull, it will likely add less flavor to the dish. Store spices in a dry, dark place in a well-sealed container.

Fermented veggies: Fermented vegetables are rich in probiotics, which may optimize gut health to better metabolize food and help your body utilize nutrients appropriately. Sauerkraut in particular contains vitamin K_2, which helps prevent calcified arteries. Sauerkraut and fermented vegetables are an easy way to add acidity to a soup, side, or main dish with a perfect amount of crunch, flavor, and gut-healthy nutrients. Look for these items in your supermarket's refrigerated section to ensure the probiotics are live and therefore active. Choose unpasteurized products because they have more health benefits. Looking for terms on the food label such as "raw," "live," "unpasteurized," and "keep refrigerated" can help verify this. Just be mindful of the salt content of these products.

No-salt-added beans and legumes: Beans and legumes are rich sources of heart-healthy vitamins and minerals, such as dietary fiber, vitamin B_6, folate, manganese, copper, and thiamine, and are a great plant-based protein alternative. Choose Tetra Paks of no-salt-added beans and legumes to reduce the salt content and BPA/BPS toxins normally found in canned beans. If you cannot find Tetra Paks, choose low-sodium canned beans with BPA-free lining and rinse the beans well before eating.

Olive oil: Olive oil is a heart-healthy monounsaturated fat that has been shown to significantly reduce blood pressure levels and decrease the risk of stroke. When purchasing olive oil, choose cold-pressed extra-virgin olive oil when possible because it is unrefined and was never treated with heat, meaning it has more health benefits. To preserve its nutrients, the olive oil should ideally be in a dark glass or metal container. Olive oil generally has a moderate-to-low smoke point and should therefore resist heat to continue to preserve its nutrients. It is a great addition to salads and, for a flavor boost, can be added after cooking. If you cannot find cold-pressed, opt for extra-virgin olive oil instead.

Tahini: Tahini is a ground sesame seed spread that contains cholesterol-reducing lignans and phytosterols—in addition to polyunsaturated and monounsaturated fats. When looking for this item, choose one with an ingredient list that only includes "sesame seeds" or "ground sesame seeds." Avoid any varieties with added oil or salt. Tahini beautifully flavors many salads, sauces, and dips to add a creamy, savory, and nutty flavor profile.

Whole grains: Whole grains such as buckwheat, quinoa, bulgur, farro, and barley can be bought in a regular bag or in the bulk-item section of many stores and can help make a dish more satisfying and filling. After a meta-analysis of 45 studies, it was concluded that eating three daily servings of whole grains can decrease the risk of heart disease by 22 percent and stroke by 12 percent. Whole grains are generally rich in dietary fiber and B vitamins—particularly thiamine, riboflavin, niacin, folate, and magnesium. If purchasing from bulk bins, be sure to store them in a container with a tight-fitting lid in a cool, dry place.

Whole oats: Whole oats are a great source of beta-glucan fiber, a specific type of soluble fiber that has been shown to lower cholesterol and LDL cholesterol significantly. They can be used in a variety of ways such as in an easy breakfast, as a binding agent in a burger or loaf, or as a flour by simply pulverizing it in the blender. Recently oats had a bad reputation for having excess amounts of glyphosate, a harmful pesticide. The way to avoid this is to aim for organic varieties instead.

Kitchen Equipment Basics

- Measuring cups and spoons
- Parchment paper (As a safe, nonstick paper, this will help reduce the amount of oil needed in a dish.)
- Kitchen utensils, such as a utilitarian chef's knife, whisk, grater, spatula, and large mixing spoon
- Mixing bowls: a small (1.5-quart), medium (2.5-quart), and a large (4-quart)
- One to two standard (14½-by-11¼-inch) cutting boards (ideally, one for vegetables and another for poultry)
- 16-by-22-inch aluminum baking sheet
- Muffin tins
- Standard 9-by-5-inch loaf pan
- 11½-inch frying pan
- 5-quart stainless steel pot
- 50- to 60-ounce high-speed blender
- 9-cup standard food processor

Easy Swaps for Processed Foods

PROCESSED FOODS TO AVOID	BETTER OPTION TO BUY	BETTER OPTION TO MAKE
Store-bought barbeque sauce	Mix 1 cup of no-salt-added tomato sauce with 2 teaspoons of low-sodium hot sauce	Barbeque Sauce (page 169)
Ranch dressing	Watered-down tahini	Tahini-Garlic Dressing (page 165)
Tartar sauce	Low-sodium aioli sauce	Tartar Sauce (page 168)
Canned, pre-packaged soups, high-sodium vegetable broths	No-salt-added vegetable soups and broths	Homemade soups (chapter 4)
Potato Chips	Low-sodium bean-based chips	Roasted Cannellini Bean "Chips" (page 152)
Instant oatmeal or packaged, sweetened oats	Old-fashioned oats or steel-cut oats	N/A
Regular crackers	Whole grain crackers with at least 3 grams of fiber	Whole Wheat Seed Crackers (page 151)
High-salt pesto sauce	N/A	Arugula-Basil Pesto (page 161)
Milk chocolate or white chocolate	85 percent vegan dark chocolate	N/A
Caesar salad dressing	Low-sodium, low-fat, yogurt-based store-bought dressing	Cashew Cream Dressing (164)

About the Recipes

These recipes are intended to make adhering to a heart-healthy diet easy by providing fast and simple meals. All of these recipes contain nutritional information for your reference to ensure the dish meets your specific needs and nutrient requirements. They also take into account individuals who need to monitor their drug nutrient interactions and who have crossover conditions.

Each recipe has two types of labels:

1 **Dietary labels:** This denotes what type of diet(s) the recipe adheres to: Vegetarian or Vegan, Low-Sodium, Low-Fat/Cholesterol, and Low-Carb. A vegan label means the dish contains no animal products or derivatives such as honey. A vegetarian label allows for dairy and consumption but excludes fish. A low-sodium dietary label means less than 150 milligrams of sodium per snack and 300 milligrams of sodium per meal. A low-fat/low-cholesterol meal means 15 grams or less of total fat per meal and 5 grams or less of total fat per snack. A low-carb diet means 30 grams or less of carbohydrates per meal, or less than 15 grams of carbohydrates per snack, after accounting for dietary fiber.

2 **Easy labels:** All meals in this book are labeled 30 Minutes or Less, One-Pot, or 5-Ingredient. This will allow you to navigate to recipes that are your preferred easy cooking method.

Each recipe will also have one of these three types of tips:

1 **Make It Easier Tip:** This tip suggests how to make the recipe faster or easier than it is already.

2 **Substitution Tip:** This tip suggests a replacement for an item, making the dish malleable for varying flavor profiles, or accommodating for specific allergies.

3 **Flavor Tip:** This tip suggests how to boost or vary the dish's flavor.

Artichoke, Basil, and Tomato Crustless Quiche

PAGE 44

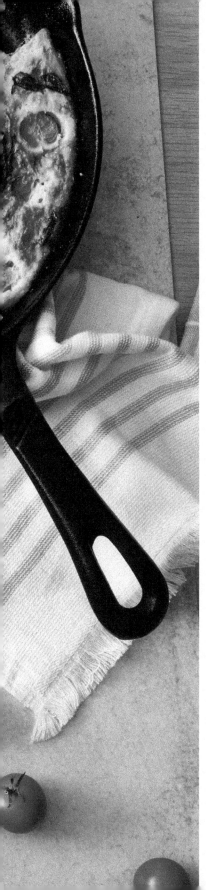

Two

BREAKFAST AND SMOOTHIES

Very Berry Kale Smoothie

SERVES 1 • PREP TIME: 5 MINUTES

LOW-CARB • LOW-FAT/LOW-CHOLESTEROL • LOW-SODIUM • VEGAN

5-INGREDIENT, 30 MINUTES OR LESS, ONE-POT

Typically, smoothies are high in sugar and lack protein. All the smoothies in this book are well balanced, featuring lean protein, healthy fat, and dietary fiber. Kale is not only high in vitamin C, vitamin K, and copper, but it has also been found to bind to bile acids in the digestive system, preventing their absorption and lowering cholesterol levels. This smoothie is refreshing, it includes antioxidant-rich berries, creaminess from the almond butter, and subtle sweetness from the dates. The soymilk adds protein to the dish, and the kale adds heart-healthy benefits without changing the taste.

1 cup frozen mixed berries

½ cup kale

2 teaspoons creamy raw unsalted almond butter

1 cup unsweetened soymilk

2 small dates or 1 Medjool date

Combine the berries, kale, almond butter, soymilk, and dates in a blender and blend for 1 minute until the ingredients are well combined. Serve immediately.

SUBSTITUTION TIP: For a grassier taste, a host of heart-healthy antioxidants, and a good source of copper, add 1 teaspoon of spirulina to the smoothie. Spirulina is a green-blue algae that has a potent antioxidant, phycocyanin, that gives it anti-inflammatory properties.

Per serving: Calories: 277; Total fat: 10g; Saturated fat: 1g; Cholesterol: 0mg; Sodium: 106mg; Potassium: 507mg; Magnesium: 78mg; Carbohydrates: 38g; Sugars: 27g; Fiber: 8.5g; Protein: 11g; Added sugar: 0g; Vitamin K: 70mcg

Ginger-Mango Smoothie

SERVES 1 • PREP TIME: 5 MINUTES

LOW-CARB • LOW-FAT/LOW-CHOLESTEROL • LOW-SODIUM • VEGETARIAN

5-INGREDIENT, 30 MINUTES OR LESS, ONE-POT

This ginger-mango smoothie is a thick yogurt-based drink with a sweet and tangy flavor. The smoothie gets its tang from fresh, anti-inflammatory ginger. Mango adds the sweetness and a healthy dose of antioxidants. The spinach adds a beautiful bright green color to the smoothie, along with a boost of dietary fiber and heart-healthy vitamins and minerals, without impacting the taste.

½ cup frozen mango

1 cup spinach

½ cup low-fat, plain
Greek yogurt

½ inch ginger, peeled

3 tablespoons water, as
needed to thin

Combine the mango, spinach, yogurt, and ginger in a blender. Blend to your desired thickness, adding water as necessary. Serve immediately.

SUBSTITUTION TIP: If you want to skip the tanginess and add a sweeter note, swap the ginger for ¼ teaspoon of ground cinnamon.

Per serving: Calories: 148; Total fat: 3g; Saturated fat: 2g; Cholesterol: 10mg; Sodium: 67mg; Potassium: 344mg; Magnesium: 41mg; Carbohydrates: 17g; Sugars: 15g; Fiber: 2g; Protein: 14g; Added sugar: 0g; Vitamin K: 149mcg

Chocolate and Peanut Butter Smoothie

SERVES 1 • PREP TIME: 10 MINUTES

LOW-CARB • LOW-FAT/LOW-CHOLESTEROL • LOW-SODIUM • VEGAN

30 MINUTES OR LESS, ONE-POT

In the mood for a hot chocolate in the morning? This chocolate and peanut butter smoothie is enhanced with a bright red, beet-fueled color that is not only beautiful but healthy—because beets have anti-inflammatory and vasodilating properties. Antioxidant-rich cacao powder is blended with silken tofu and sweetened with bananas, peanut butter, and earthy beets to form a velvety smooth, protein-rich, well-balanced breakfast smoothie. Enjoy it cold or warm it up for 1 to 2 minutes for a hot chocolate breakfast.

1 medium beet, peeled and quartered

1 tablespoon unsweetened cacao powder

2 teaspoons unsalted raw peanut butter

½ medium banana

3 ounces silken tofu

1 cup unsweetened almond milk

Combine the beet, cacao powder, peanut butter, banana, tofu, and almond milk in a blender and blend for 1 to 2 minutes until well combined. Serve immediately.

FLAVOR TIP: Add ½ teaspoon of vanilla extract if you want to add a floral, woodsy taste and aromatic note.

Per serving: Calories: 261; Total fat: 11g; Saturated fat: 2g; Cholesterol: 0mg; Sodium: 268mg; Potassium: 1075mg; Magnesium: 109mg; Carbohydrates: 30g; Sugars: 15g; Fiber: 6.5g; Protein: 13g; Added sugar: 0g; Vitamin K: 3mcg

Berry, Walnut, and Cinnamon Quinoa Bowl

SERVES 2 • PREP TIME: 5 MINUTES • COOK TIME: 15 MINUTES

LOW-CARB • LOW-FAT/LOW-CHOLESTEROL • LOW-SODIUM • VEGAN

5-INGREDIENT, 30 MINUTES OR LESS, ONE-POT

Quinoa, pronounced *keen-wah*, is technically a seed that's lumped into the whole grain category because it's too small to mill. Incans called it *chisaya mama*, the "mother of all grains." Quinoa has a fluffy, creamy texture that picks up flavors well. In this bowl, airy quinoa is combined with aromatic cinnamon, crunchy toasted walnuts, and sweet strawberries to comfort, nourish, and satiate you. If you are allergic to nuts, substitute the walnuts for sunflower seeds instead.

½ cup quinoa

1 cup unsweetened almond milk

1 teaspoon cinnamon, plus more for coating

10 raw walnuts

1 cup strawberries, sliced

1. Preheat the oven to 425°F and line a baking sheet with parchment paper. In a medium pot, bring the quinoa, almond milk, and cinnamon to a boil.

2. Lower the heat to a simmer and cover for 12 minutes, or until the almond milk has been absorbed.

3. Put the walnuts and a dash of cinnamon onto the prepared baking sheet and bake for 5 minutes until lightly golden.

4. In a serving bowl, combine the quinoa and walnuts, and top with the strawberries. (When storing, put the quinoa only in the refrigerator for up to 1 week. Add the walnuts and strawberries when ready to eat.)

MAKE IT EASIER TIP: Instead of toasting only 10 walnuts, toast several servings and store the walnuts in an airtight container until you need them.

Per serving: Calories: 268; Total fat: 11g; Saturated fat: 1g; Cholesterol: 0mg; Sodium: 88mg; Potassium: 486mg; Magnesium: 119mg; Carbohydrates: 36g; Sugars: 7g; Fiber: 6g; Protein: 9g; Added sugar: 0g; Vitamin K: 2mcg

Pumpkin-Pecan Greek Yogurt Overnight Oatmeal

SERVES 1 • PREP TIME: 5 MINUTES, PLUS OVERNIGHT TO CHILL

LOW-CARB • LOW-FAT/LOW-CHOLESTEROL • LOW-SODIUM • VEGETARIAN

30 MINUTES OR LESS, ONE-POT

Oatmeal is usually made in one of three ways: Taking oat groats and rolling them (rolled oats), crushing them (quick oats), or "steel-cutting" them (steel-cut oats). Pairing oats with vitamin C may help increase their ability to reduce inflammation, and this dish does just that by adding in pumpkin. This pumpkin-pecan oatmeal is a breakfast for champions, evoking feelings of fall. It is well balanced with protein, complex carbohydrates, and dietary fiber, and makes an easy grab-and-go meal.

½ cup fat-free or low-fat plain Greek yogurt

¼ cup oats

¼ cup unsweetened almond milk

¼ teaspoon vanilla extract

½ cup no-sugar-added canned pumpkin puree

¼ teaspoon pumpkin spice

2 teaspoons unsalted raw pecans, chopped

1. In a Mason jar or medium container, put the yogurt, oats, almond milk, vanilla, pumpkin, and pumpkin spice. Mix the ingredients well.

2. Store overnight in the refrigerator. Mix the ingredients again in the morning and top with the pecans. Leftovers are good for 3 days; the more the oatmeal sits, the softer the oats become.

SUBSTITUTION TIP: For a creamy texture, use rolled oats. For a chewier texture, swap for quick-cooking steel-cut oats.

Per serving: Calories: 227; Total fat: 4.6g; Saturated fat: 0.5g; Cholesterol: 6mg; Sodium: 93mg; Potassium: 402mg; Magnesium: 79mg; Carbohydrates: 29g; Sugars: 9g; Fiber: 5g; Protein: 17g; Added sugar: 0g; Vitamin K: 21mcg

Chocolate-Oatmeal Loaf

SERVES 6 • PREP TIME: 10 MINUTES • COOK TIME: 20 MINUTES

LOW-CARB • LOW-FAT/LOW-CHOLESTEROL • LOW-SODIUM • VEGAN

30 MINUTES OR LESS

This spongy, chocolatey, and flavorful recipe uses ground flaxseed and soymilk to hold the mixture together. You can buy flaxseed whole and grind it yourself or buy it ground and refrigerate it once opened to prevent it from losing its heart-healthy benefits. Cacao powder, pure maple syrup, and almond butter give this loaf a nutty, chocolaty taste with a subtle hint of sweetness.

Nonstick avocado oil cooking spray

2 tablespoons ground flaxseed

5 tablespoons unsweetened organic soymilk

1¼ cups rolled oats

1 teaspoon baking powder

2 tablespoons unsweetened cacao powder

1 teaspoon cinnamon

1 tablespoon pure maple syrup

1 banana, mashed

2 tablespoons unsalted raw almond butter

1. Preheat the oven to 400°F. Spray a standard (8½-by-4½-by-2½-inch) loaf pan with cooking spray or grease it with 1 teaspoon of oil spread equally on the sides. Place the pan in the oven.

2. In a small mixing bowl, mix the flaxseed and soymilk and let the mixture sit for 5 minutes, until it congeals.

3. In a large mixing bowl, combine the oats, baking powder, cacao powder, and cinnamon and mix well. In a small mixing bowl, combine the maple syrup, banana, almond butter, and flaxseed mixture and mix well. Add the dry ingredients into the wet ingredients until well combined.

4. Carefully take the loaf pan out of the oven and pour the mixture into it. Bake for 20 minutes, or until a fork inserted into the middle of the loaf comes out clean. This loaf is best served warm. Store in the refrigerator covered for up to 1 week. To rewarm, heat in the microwave in 15-second increments until warm.

FLAVOR TIP: Break apart ¼ of a bar of 85 percent dark chocolate and spread evenly on top of the loaf before you bake. It makes for a delicious breakfast oozing with chocolate.

Per serving: Calories: 152; Total fat: 6g; Saturated fat: 1g; Cholesterol: 0mg; Sodium: 89mg; Potassium: 195mg; Magnesium: 46mg; Carbohydrates: 21g; Sugars: 5g; Fiber: 4g; Protein: 5g; Added sugar: 2g; Vitamin K: 1mcg

Kefir Parfait with Chia Berry Jam

SERVES 2 • PREP TIME: 10 MINUTES

LOW-CARB • LOW-FAT/LOW-CHOLESTEROL • LOW-SODIUM • VEGETARIAN

5-INGREDIENT, 30 MINUTES OR LESS, ONE-POT

Kefir is a tart, fermented milk beverage; think drinkable yogurt. It originated from the Caucasus Mountains and comes from the word *Keyir*, a Turkish word meaning "feeling good," which I translate as making your gut feel good! Kefir is loaded with probiotics (61 strains!) that help the gut microbiome better absorb nutrients. Pairing kefir with chia and berries creates a well-balanced meal that tastes delicious, smooth, and tart.

12 ounces low-fat kefir

4 tablespoons Chia Berry Jam (page 171)

Into each of two serving bowls, place half of the kefir and 2 tablespoons of chia jam and dig in!

FLAVOR TIP: To sweeten the dish, add 1 teaspoon of pure maple syrup. Pure maple syrup has 24 antioxidants and the mineral manganese, which plays a positive role in blood clotting and reduces inflammation. Avoid syrups with added sugars or high-fructose corn syrup.

SERVING TIP: If you have extra time or want to pretty this dish up for a guest, layer 2 ounces of kefir with ½ tablespoon of chia jam, alternating until 2 layers are made per person.

Per serving: Calories: 113; Total fat: 3g; Saturated fat: 1g; Cholesterol: 9mg; Sodium: 71mg; Potassium: 279mg; Magnesium: 20mg; Carbohydrates: 13g; Sugars: 10g; Fiber: 3g; Protein: 8g; Added sugar: 0g; Vitamin K: 5mcg

Greek Yogurt Topped with Turmeric-Spiced Almonds and Pumpkin Seeds

SERVES 2 • PREP TIME: 5 MINUTES • COOK TIME: 10 MINUTES

LOW-CARB • LOW-FAT/LOW-CHOLESTEROL • LOW-SODIUM • VEGETARIAN

5-INGREDIENT, 30 MINUTES OR LESS, ONE-POT

Flavoring almonds and pumpkin seeds with a turmeric and cinnamon spice mix will fill your home with a calming aroma. Turmeric's active ingredient is curcumin, which is poorly absorbed by the body. However, pairing it with black pepper increases its absorption by 2,000 percent. I add black pepper to give your body a host of anti-inflammatory turmeric benefits, but trust me, there won't be any peppery taste in this dish. Pair the spiced nuts with Greek yogurt and perhaps a high-fiber fruit for a delicious, filling, and satisfying breakfast.

¼ teaspoon ground turmeric

¼ teaspoon cinnamon powder

⅛ teaspoon freshly ground black pepper

¼ cup raw almonds, sliced

¼ cup raw pumpkin seeds

2 cups fat-free or low-fat plain Greek yogurt

1. Preheat the oven to 425°F. Line a baking sheet with parchment paper.

2. On the baking sheet pan, mix the turmeric, cinnamon, and black pepper with the almonds and pumpkin seeds. Spread them out once thoroughly mixed, so they do not overlap.

3. Bake for 5 to 8 minutes, until golden brown and fragrant.

4. To serve, fill each serving bowl with 1 cup of yogurt and top with the nut and seed mixture. Store nuts in an airtight container in the refrigerator for up to 5 days.

FLAVOR TIP: For more dietary fiber, antioxidants, a heart-healthy boost, *and* a delectable balance of sweet and tart, add 1 cup of blackberries per bowl.

Per serving: Calories: 310; Total fat: 15g; Saturated fat: 2g; Cholesterol: 12mg; Sodium: 91mg; Potassium: 571mg; Magnesium: 146mg; Carbohydrates: 15g; Sugars: 9g; Fiber: 3g; Protein: 32g; Added sugar: 0g; Vitamin K: 2mcg

Chia Seed, Blueberry, and Yogurt Pancakes

SERVES 2 • PREP TIME: 5 MINUTES • COOK TIME: 9 MINUTES
LOW-FAT/LOW-CHOLESTEROL • LOW-SODIUM • VEGETARIAN

30 MINUTES OR LESS, ONE-POT

This recipe is a family original that my husband makes for our kids on Sunday mornings. Most pancakes are high in simple carbohydrates and lack protein. These fluffy, moist, and colorful complex carbohydrates (oats and blueberries), lean protein (yogurt), and healthy fat (chia seeds) for a more well-rounded breakfast. These pancakes are fluffy and moist from the yogurt, and juicy and colorful from the beautiful blueberries. These can be made ahead of time and stored in the refrigerator for 3 or 4 days.

1 cup rolled oats

1 cup blueberries

3 tablespoons fat-free, plain Greek yogurt

¼ cup unsweetened soymilk

1 tablespoon chia seeds

1 egg

½ teaspoon cinnamon

2 teaspoons avocado oil

1. In a medium mixing bowl, mix the oats, blueberries, yogurt, soymilk, chia seeds, egg, and cinnamon until a doughy consistency forms.

2. In a large skillet, heat the oil over medium-low heat and add the batter. Make either one large pancake that covers the entire pan or make smaller individual pancakes.

3. Cook for 4 to 5 minutes. Once the edges are brown, flip the pancake. To make it easier to flip, you can cut the larger pancake into 4 sections and flip them individually.

4. Cook on the opposite side for 1 or 2 minutes, until the pancake is no longer doughy. Serve warm and top with your favorite toppings.

FLAVOR TIP: Top with 1 teaspoon of your favorite nut butter and 1 tablespoon of Chia Berry Jam (page 171) for a delicious "syrup" instead of traditional high-sugar pancake syrup.

Per serving: Calories: 328; Total fat: 12g; Saturated fat: 2g; Cholesterol: 83mg; Sodium: 54mg; Potassium: 304mg; Magnesium: 70mg; Carbohydrates: 43g; Sugars: 10g; Fiber: 9g; Protein: 13g; Added sugar: 0g; Vitamin K: 15mcg

Swiss Chard and Tzatziki Dip on Whole Wheat Toast

SERVES 2 • PREP TIME: 10 MINUTES • COOK TIME: 10 MINUTES

LOW-CARB • LOW-FAT/LOW-CHOLESTEROL • LOW-SODIUM • VEGETARIAN

5-INGREDIENT, 30 MINUTES OR LESS, ONE-POT

Swiss chard is siblings with beets and spinach, and they have a couple things in common: Swiss chard's stems have a sweet beet-like taste and its leaves taste like spinach. Swiss chard is full of heart-healthy vitamins, such as vitamin C, magnesium, and potassium. Sautéing the chard stalks with their leaves and the caramelized onion imparts a sweet-and-savory flavor that perfectly accompanies a refreshing yogurt dip atop a toasted, crispy whole wheat slice of bread.

1 teaspoon avocado oil

1 small onion, chopped

2 garlic cloves, thinly sliced

1 bunch Swiss chard, stems diced and leaves chopped, divided

2 slices low-sodium whole wheat bread

1 cup Tzatziki Dip (page 167)

1. In a medium pot, heat the oil over medium-low heat and add the onion, garlic, and Swiss chard stems. Heat for 5 minutes, until the onions become translucent and the chard stalks bleed red into the dish.

2. Add the chard leaves and cover for 5 minutes, until the leaves are wilted and the dish is fragrant.

3. Meanwhile, toast the bread until crisp. Place it on a serving plate and top each slice of bread with 1 cup of cooked Swiss chard and ½ cup of the dip.

MAKE IT EASIER TIP: Cut 15 minutes out of this recipe by prepping the dip and greens beforehand and assembling it in the morning. Both the tzatziki and greens can be stored in the refrigerator for up to 5 days.

Per serving: Calories: 214; Total fat: 4g; Saturated fat: 1g; Cholesterol: 5mg; Sodium: 111mg; Potassium: 603mg; Magnesium: 95mg; Carbohydrates: 28g; Sugars: 8g; Fiber: 4g; Protein: 18g; Added sugar: 0g; Vitamin K: 605mcg

Apple, Cinnamon, and Cardamom Whole Grain Breakfast Muffins

SERVES 8 • PREP TIME: 15 MINUTES • COOK TIME: 15 MINUTES
LOW-CARB • LOW-FAT/LOW-CHOLESTEROL • LOW-SODIUM • VEGETARIAN

30 MINUTES OR LESS

Muffins are typically high in refined sugars and lack satiating protein, causing a sugar spike and hunger shortly after eating. This recipe packs in complex carbohydrates, dietary fiber, and protein to keep your blood sugar balanced and your stomach happy. It is soft, spongy, and deliciously sweetened with loads of apples, a couple chopped dates, and cinnamon and cardamom. Enjoy these warm so you can enjoy the apple pie–like scent, texture, and taste. Try swapping the cardamom for pumpkin spice, which is typically a combination of cinnamon, nutmeg, and cloves.

1¾ cups whole wheat flour

½ teaspoon baking powder

2 tablespoons cinnamon

1½ teaspoons cardamom

3 whole eggs

¾ cup low-fat, plain Greek yogurt

¾ cup unsweetened applesauce

3 large dates, chopped

3 cups Gala apples, peeled, cored, and cut into bite-size pieces

1. Preheat the oven to 400°F. Line a muffin tin with 8 muffin liners.

2. In a medium mixing bowl, combine the flour, baking powder, cinnamon, and cardamom.

3. In a large mixing bowl, combine the eggs, Greek yogurt, applesauce, and dates.

4. Using either a spatula or hand whisk, fold half of the dry ingredients into the full bowl of wet ingredients, then fold in the other half. Stir in the apple pieces until evenly distributed throughout the batter.

5. Divide the batter evenly into the prepared muffin tin. Bake for 15 minutes, or until a toothpick inserted into the center of the muffins comes out clean. Store in an airtight container in the refrigerator for up to a week. Warm in the microwave in 15-second increments.

Per serving: Calories: 168; Total fat: 3g; Saturated fat: 1g; Cholesterol: 63mg; Sodium: 63mg; Potassium: 214mg; Magnesium: 45mg; Carbohydrates: 30g; Sugars: 8g; Fiber: 5g; Protein: 8g; Added sugar: 0g; Vitamin K: 2mcg

Black Bean and Avocado Breakfast Tacos

SERVES 2 • PREP TIME: 5 MINUTES • COOK TIME: 5 MINUTES (WITH EGG)

LOW-FAT/LOW-CHOLESTEROL • LOW-SODIUM • VEGAN

30 MINUTES OR LESS, ONE-POT

This dish combines ripe, creamy, and heart-healthy avocado with juicy mango, tangy lime, and tender black beans for a well-balanced, refreshing breakfast. Avocados are a rich source of folate, potassium, and both types of dietary fiber, which may help reduce LDL cholesterol levels, improve blood sugar levels, and assist with weight management. Add a poached egg, if you please, for an extra-oozy yolk explosion upon your first bite.

1 cup canned black beans, drained and rinsed

½ ripe avocado, diced

½ mango, diced

2 tablespoons lime juice (1 lime)

¼ cup chopped fresh cilantro

1 tablespoon rice vinegar (optional)

1 egg, poached (optional)

2 low-sodium whole wheat taco-size tortillas

1. In a medium mixing bowl, combine the black beans, avocado, mango, lime juice, and cilantro. Mix well.

2. *If adding the egg:* Fill a medium pot with water halfway and bring to a boil. Add the rice vinegar. Crack the egg into a small mixing bowl. Reduce the heat to a simmer. Stir the water with a slotted spoon to create a vortex, drop the egg inside, and cook for 3 minutes, until the white has set. Remove carefully with the slotted spoon and place on a paper towel.

3. Spread the black bean mixture on a tortilla, place the poached egg on top (if using), and serve. The black bean mixture can be stored in an airtight container for up to 3 days.

MAKE IT EASIER TIP: This dish is one-pot and made in 5 minutes if you skip the egg. If you would like the poached egg but don't have time, consider preparing it the night before. You can store poached eggs for up to 2 days in the refrigerator, but they're best when you only store them overnight. Prepare the poached egg as above and have an ice bath ready for when it's done; store it in an airtight container filled with cool water. To serve, simmer the egg in a pot of water for about a minute.

Per serving: Calories: 294; Total fat: 7g; Saturated fat: 2g; Cholesterol: 0mg; Sodium: 130mg; Potassium: 684mg; Magnesium: 66mg; Carbohydrates: 50g; Sugars: 13g; Fiber: 14g; Protein: 10g; Added sugar: 0g; Vitamin K: 11mcg

Chickpea and Brussels Sprouts Hash

SERVES 2 • PREP TIME: 10 MINUTES • COOK TIME: 10 MINUTES

LOW-CARB • LOW-FAT/LOW-CHOLESTEROL • LOW-SODIUM • VEGAN

5-INGREDIENT, 30 MINUTES OR LESS

This chickpea and Brussels sprouts hash is both savory and delicious, providing a palatable, nutritious, and satiating breakfast meal. Chickpeas are one of the highest plant-based protein sources of vitamin B_6. Chickpeas may also help with weight management and blood sugar control. This dish is flavored with nutritional yeast, which has a cheesy and nutty flavor and is rich in protein and fortified with B vitamins, particularly B_{12}, which is otherwise only found in animal protein.

½ cup canned chickpeas, reserving 2 tablespoons packing water

2 tablespoons water

¼ teaspoon freshly ground black pepper

1 tablespoon nutritional yeast

1 teaspoon chia seeds

2 teaspoons avocado oil

1 scallion, finely chopped

1 cup shaved Brussels sprouts

1. In a blender, put the chickpeas, reserved packing water, water, pepper, and nutritional yeast. Blend for 1 to 2 minutes, until the ingredients are well combined but the chickpeas still have some texture. Add the chia seeds to the mixture and let sit for about 5 minutes.

2. In a medium saucepan, heat the oil on medium heat for about 1 minute, until the pan is hot. Then add the chickpea mixture and cook for about 3 minutes, stirring occasionally. Using a spatula, chop the formed mixture in the pan to resemble a hash. Add in the scallion and cook for 1 more minute, until the chickpea mixture is lightly browned.

3. Add the Brussels sprouts, cover, and cook for 2 minutes, until the sprouts become slightly wilted. Divide the mixture in half and serve. Store in the refrigerator in an airtight container for up to 3 days.

SUBSTITUTION TIP: To have a more subtle and milder onion flavor, swap the scallion for chives.

Per serving: Calories: 142; Total fat: 7g; Saturated fat: 1g; Cholesterol: 0mg; Sodium: 113mg; Potassium: 145mg; Magnesium: 17mg; Carbohydrates: 16g; Sugars: 3g; Fiber: 6g; Protein: 7g; Added sugar: 0g; Vitamin K: 135mcg

Buckwheat, Asparagus, and Tomato Savory Breakfast Bowl

SERVES 2 • PREP TIME: 10 MINUTES • COOK TIME: 20 MINUTES
LOW-FAT/LOW-CHOLESTEROL • LOW-SODIUM • VEGAN

5-INGREDIENT, 30 MINUTES OR LESS

Despite its name, buckwheat is a gluten-free seed that is considered a whole grain. Buckwheat is high in soluble fibers that have been shown to reduce blood sugar levels, meaning you'll avoid a morning sugar spike. Buckwheat has an earthy taste, and this dish pairs it with smashed garlic to add flavor. The creamy buckwheat, sautéed asparagus, and blistered tomatoes make a savory and comforting breakfast meal. Squeeze a lemon on top for a bright citrus finish.

½ cup buckwheat

3 cups water

2 garlic cloves, smashed

2 teaspoons avocado oil

2 cups asparagus (about 20 spears), sliced

1 cup cherry tomatoes

1 teaspoon Mediterranean Seasoning Rub Blend (page 159)

1. In a medium saucepan, bring the buckwheat, water, and garlic to a boil, then reduce the heat to low and cover for about 15 minutes, until the buckwheat groats are opened, exposing a creamy white texture, and the majority of the water has cooked out. Do not drain the water; it will soak into and thicken the mixture as it sits.

2. In the meantime, in a medium skillet, heat the oil, asparagus, cherry tomatoes, and the spice blend on medium-low heat. Mix well and cook for 4 to 6 minutes, until the tomatoes are blistered and the asparagus is fork-tender.

3. Add the asparagus and tomatoes to the buckwheat. Mix well, divide into two servings, and serve or store in an airtight container in the refrigerator for up to 5 days.

MAKE IT EASIER TIP: Prep the buckwheat the night before and add in leftover seasoned, roasted veggies the next day for an easy-to-assemble breakfast.

Per serving: Calories: 232; Total fat: 6g; Saturated fat: 1g; Cholesterol: 0mg; Sodium: 13mg; Potassium: 636mg; Magnesium: 121mg; Carbohydrates: 41g; Sugars: 6g; Fiber: 9g; Protein: 9g; Added sugar: 0g; Vitamin K: 76mcg

Fluffy Veggie Egg Omelet

SERVES 1 • PREP TIME: 10 MINUTES • COOK TIME: 10 MINUTES

LOW-CARB • LOW-FAT/LOW-CHOLESTEROL • LOW-SODIUM • VEGETARIAN

30 MINUTES OR LESS, ONE-POT

These fluffy eggs are jam-packed with flavor from the aromatic Mediterranean Spice Blend, caramelized onions, sweet and crunchy orange bell peppers, and wilted spinach. If you're avoiding whole eggs, swap out the 2 whole eggs for 3 egg whites. This breakfast meal can be enjoyed as is or paired with a whole wheat, high-fiber crispbread or Whole Wheat Seed Crackers (page 151).

1 teaspoon avocado oil

1 small onion, diced

½ cup orange bell pepper, diced

2 medium eggs

2 egg whites

2 tablespoons water

1 cup packed fresh spinach

¼ teaspoon Mediterranean Seasoning Rub Blend (page 159)

1. In a medium pan, heat the oil over medium heat. Add the onions and cook until translucent, about 1 minute. Add the bell peppers and cook for an additional 2 minutes.

2. Meanwhile, in a small mixing bowl, combine the eggs, egg whites, and water and whisk together until well combined.

3. Add the spinach and spice blend to the medium pan. Stir and cook for 1 minute, until the spinach is wilted. Add the eggs and cook, covered, for 3 minutes until the edges are lightly browned. Uncover, flip, and cook for 1 to 2 minutes more, until the eggs are cooked through. Serve on a plate.

MAKE IT EASIER TIP: For an easy grab-and-go option, batch-cook this recipe by tripling the ingredients. Divide the ingredients equally in the cups of a muffin tin and bake at 350°F for 20 to 25 minutes. You'll get delicious egg muffin frittatas you can store in the refrigerator or even the freezer and easily pop out as a breakfast or snack. If frozen, wrap the frittatas in a damp paper towel and microwave in 15-second increments until warm.

Per serving: Calories: 263; Total fat: 4g; Saturated fat: 3g; Cholesterol: 328mg; Sodium: 237mg; Potassium: 646mg; Magnesium: 56mg; Carbohydrates: 8g; Sugars: 5g; Fiber: 2g; Protein: 20g; Added sugar: 0g; Vitamin K: 228mcg

Tofu Shakshuka

SERVES 4 • PREP TIME: 10 MINUTES • COOK TIME: 15 MINUTES
LOW-CARB • LOW-FAT/LOW-CHOLESTEROL • LOW-SODIUM • VEGAN

30 MINUTES OR LESS, ONE-POT

Shakshuka is an Israeli dish that means "all mixed up" and is typically made with eggs cooked in tomato sauce. This rendition swaps eggs for tofu, which soaks up the delicious tomato, red pepper, onion, and basil flavors. This dish can easily be accompanied with whole wheat bread or ½ cup of a whole grain of your choice to pick up the mouth-watering juices.

2 teaspoons avocado oil

1 large onion, diced

1 large red bell pepper, diced

2 large tomatoes, diced

3 tablespoons double-concentrated tomato paste

½ cup water

1 (14-ounce) package firm tofu, cut into 1-inch-thick square pieces

4 heaping tablespoons chopped fresh basil

2 teaspoons Mediterranean Seasoning Rub Blend (page 159)

1. In a large pot, heat the oil over medium heat. Add the onion, bell pepper, and tomatoes and cook for about 2 minutes, until the onions are translucent. Add the tomato paste and water to the pot, stir, and cover. Cook for 5 minutes, until the peppers are fork-tender and the tomatoes are soft.

2. Add the tofu, basil, and spice blend and combine well with other ingredients. Cook, covered, for another 5 to 10 minutes, until fragrant, stirring occasionally. Divide among four plates and serve, or store in an airtight container in the refrigerator for up to 5 days.

SUBSTITUTION TIP: Easily replace the tofu with 2 cups of whole chickpeas.

Per serving: Calories: 227; Total fat: 12g; Saturated fat: 2g; Cholesterol: 0mg; Sodium: 87mg; Potassium: 625mg; Magnesium: 80mg; Carbohydrates: 15g; Sugars: 8g; Fiber: 5g; Protein: 20g; Added sugar: 0g; Vitamin K: 22mcg

Artichoke, Basil, and Tomato Crustless Quiche

SERVES 4 • PREP TIME: 10 MINUTES • COOK TIME: 20 MINUTES, PLUS 10 MINUTES TO COOL
LOW-CARB • LOW-FAT/LOW-CHOLESTEROL • LOW-SODIUM • VEGETARIAN

30 MINUTES OR LESS, ONE-POT

Artichokes are a herbaceous Mediterranean plant with a mild taste, similar to asparagus. Frozen artichokes have no salt added and easily defrost in a pinch. This crustless artichoke quiche is baked in a cast-iron skillet with a sweet, peppery, basil-and-tomato flavor and a creamy ricotta filling. This is an easy meal-prep dish, allowing you to have four deliciously balanced breakfasts ready with a quick 30-second warm-up.

2 cups artichoke hearts, finely chopped

⅓ cup chopped fresh basil

1 cup cherry tomatoes, halved

¾ teaspoon freshly ground black pepper

¼ cup part-skim ricotta cheese

4 whole eggs

8 egg whites

Avocado oil spray

1. Preheat the oven to 400°F.

2. In a large mixing bowl, mix the artichoke hearts, basil, tomatoes, pepper, ricotta cheese, whole eggs, and egg whites, and combine well.

3. Spray a large oven-safe dish with cooking spray (or evenly grease it with 1 teaspoon of avocado oil). Pour the mixture into a cast-iron skillet or oven-safe pan and bake in the oven for 15 minutes at 400°F, then increase the heat to 425°F for an additional 5 minutes, until the eggs are baked through and the edges are slightly browned. After cooled for at least 10 minutes, divide into 4 or 8 even pieces and serve, or store in the refrigerator for 5 to 7 days.

FLAVOR TIP: To create a flavorful crust, mix about ½ cup of almond flour with ¼ cup of water until it's a paste with no excess water. Add 1 minced fresh garlic clove and 1 teaspoon of dried basil. Mix well and line the bottom of the cast-iron skillet with the mixture. Bake it in the oven for about 5 minutes before adding the quiche ingredients.

Per serving: Calories: 160; Total fat: 6g; Saturated fat: 2g; Cholesterol: 169mg; Sodium: 250mg; Potassium: 585mg; Magnesium: 71mg; Carbohydrates: 8g; Sugars: 2g; Fiber: 4g; Protein: 17g; Added sugar: 0g; Vitamin K: 23mcg

No-Bake Carrot Cake Breakfast Bites

SERVES 4 • PREP TIME: 10 MINUTES, PLUS 10 MINUTES TO CHILL

LOW-CARB • LOW-FAT/LOW-CHOLESTEROL • LOW-SODIUM • VEGAN

5-INGREDIENT, 30 MINUTES OR LESS, ONE-POT

Among common fruits and vegetables, carrots have the highest amount of beta-carotene, a potent antioxidant—carotenoid is actually named after the carrot! The deeper a carrot's color, the more beta-carotene it has. In this dish, carrots are matched with dates, oats, walnuts, and pumpkin spice for a sweet-and-fresh carrot cake taste.

1 cup shredded carrots (about 2 medium carrots)

4 Medjool dates

¾ cup rolled oats

¼ cup raw walnuts

½ teaspoon pumpkin spice

1. Line a baking sheet with parchment paper.

2. In a large mixing bowl for a food processor, blend the carrots, dates, oats, walnuts, and pumpkin spice for 3 minutes until the consistency is doughy, scraping down the sides halfway through.

3. Form the mixture into bite-size balls, place on the prepared baking sheet, and put the sheet into the freezer for 10 minutes, until the breakfast bites maintain their shape. Store in an airtight container in the refrigerator for up to 5 days.

MAKE IT EASIER TIP: Instead of creating breakfast bites, line a baking sheet with parchment paper, spread the doughy mixture out evenly to about 1-inch thick, and cut into 6 bars. Place the baking sheet into the freezer for 30 to 45 minutes until the bars set. Now you have no-bake carrot bars for breakfast on the go!

Per serving (3 balls): Calories: 178; Total fat: 5g; Saturated fat: 1g; Cholesterol: 0mg; Sodium: 22mg; Potassium: 349mg; Magnesium: 48mg; Carbohydrates: 32g; Sugars: 18g; Fiber: 4g; Protein: 4g; Added sugar: 0g; Vitamin K: 5mcg

Quinoa, Edamame, and Carrot Salad with Ginger-Sesame Dressing

PAGE 56

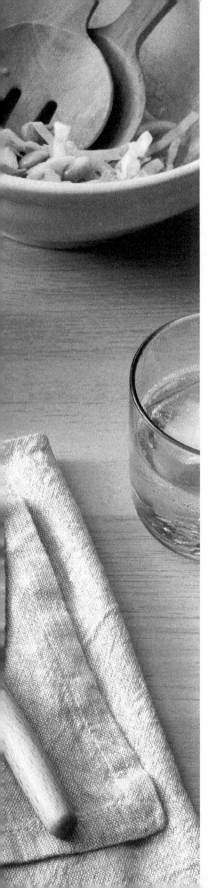

Three

SALADS

Radish, Cucumber, and Mint Salad

SERVES 2 • PREP TIME: 10 MINUTES

LOW-CARB • LOW-FAT/LOW-CHOLESTEROL • LOW-SODIUM • VEGAN

5-INGREDIENT, 30 MINUTES OR LESS, ONE-POT

This crunchy, fresh salad is colorful and delicious. The radishes have a spicy, crisp taste that pairs with cucumber and fresh mint for a cooling effect. They are married by a subtle rice vinegar dressing that brings the whole dish together. Radishes are particularly high in lignin, a type of insoluble fiber that helps your digestive system and may lower your LDL cholesterol levels.

2 tablespoons extra-virgin olive oil

2 teaspoons rice vinegar

¼ cup shredded mint, or 4 teaspoons dried

6 medium red radishes (about 1 radish bunch), cut into rounds

1 large English cucumber, cut into rounds

Freshly ground black pepper

1. In a large mixing bowl, combine the olive oil, rice vinegar, and mint and mix well.

2. Add the radishes and cucumber and combine until everything is well incorporated. Season with the pepper and serve immediately.

FLAVOR TIP: For a sweeter radish, swap red radishes for watermelon radishes. This will also add a pop of color since they are green on the outside but pink inside.

Per serving: Calories: 140; Total fat: 14g; Saturated fat: 2g; Cholesterol: 0mg; Sodium: 9mg; Potassium: 262mg; Magnesium: 8mg; Carbohydrates: 4g; Sugars: 2g; Fiber: 2g; Protein: 2g; Added sugar: 0g; Vitamin K: 8mcg

Warm Balsamic Beet Salad with Sunflower Seeds

SERVES 2 • PREP TIME: 10 MINUTES • COOK TIME: 15 MINUTES

LOW-CARB • LOW-FAT/LOW-CHOLESTEROL • LOW-SODIUM • VEGAN

5-INGREDIENT, 30 MINUTES OR LESS, ONE-POT

The entire beet—including the bulbs and the stems—is this dish's star. Beets have so many heart-healthy compounds, from their anthocyanin compounds that give them their beautiful color to its high nitrate content that helps decrease inflammation and improve blood flow. This salad uses the whole beet plant to create a salad bursting with flavor when paired with balsamic vinegar and sunflower seeds.

2 teaspoons avocado oil

3 medium whole beets, including greens and roots, chopped, divided

1 tablespoon balsamic vinegar

1 tablespoon sunflower seeds

1. In a medium pot, heat the oil over medium heat for about 2 minutes.

2. Add the beet roots and cook, covered, for 5 to 7 minutes, until they are fork-tender but not soft.

3. Add the beet greens to the pan and cook for an additional 5 to 7 minutes, uncovered, until the beets are tender and the greens are wilted.

4. In a large mixing bowl, combine balsamic vinegar, sunflower seeds, and the beet mixture and serve or store in an airtight container in the refrigerator for up to 3 days.

FLAVOR TIP: Add 2 minced garlic cloves to the diced beets in step 2 for added flavor.

Per serving: Calories: 111; Total fat: 5g; Saturated fat: 1g; Cholesterol: 0mg; Sodium: 141mg; Potassium: 554mg; Magnesium: 44mg; Carbohydrates: 14g; Sugars: 10g; Fiber: 6g; Protein: 4g; Added sugar: 0g; Vitamin K: 228mcg

Tahini, Broccoli, and Carrot Slaw

SERVES 2 • PREP TIME: 10 MINUTES

LOW-CARB • LOW-FAT/LOW-CHOLESTEROL • LOW-SODIUM • VEGAN

5-INGREDIENT, 30 MINUTES OR LESS, ONE-POT

Tahini is made from ground sesame seeds and has a creamy texture. It originated in Persia where it was called *ardeh*. When purchasing tahini, look for a product whose only ingredient is sesame seeds. It should naturally separate; just store it upside down to easily stir the oil into the paste well before using. This tahini-based salad dressing adds a creamy, nutty, and garlicky flavor to crunchy broccoli and carrot strips.

2 cups broccoli slaw, cut into matchsticks

2 cups carrot slaw, cut into matchsticks

2 tablespoons Tahini-Garlic Dressing (page 165)

In a large mixing bowl, combine the broccoli slaw, carrot slaw, and dressing and divide into two serving bowls.

MAKE IT EASIER TIP: Buy pre-chopped broccoli slaw, cabbage slaw, Brussels sprouts slaw, or carrot slaw and mix with a previously made batch of Tahini-Garlic Dressing to make the salad without much prep. Just assemble and eat!

Per serving: Calories: 140; Total fat: 6g; Saturated fat: 1g; Cholesterol: 0mg; Sodium: 95mg; Potassium: 301mg; Magnesium: 11mg; Carbohydrates: 14g; Sugars: 8g; Fiber: 4g; Protein: 4g; Added sugar: 0g; Vitamin K: 107mcg

Red Cabbage and Apple Salad with Apple Cider Vinegar and Honey Dressing

SERVES 2 • PREP TIME: 10 MINUTES

LOW-CARB • LOW-FAT/LOW-CHOLESTEROL • LOW-SODIUM • VEGETARIAN

5-INGREDIENT, 30 MINUTES OR LESS, ONE-POT

This delicious salad is made with a crunchy red cabbage base paired with tart, crisp Granny Smith apple slices. It is dressed with apple cider vinegar and a touch of honey to bring it all together. When choosing an apple cider vinegar, look for one that includes the "mother," which is the sediment that sits on the bottom of the bottle of unrefined, unpasteurized, unfiltered apple cider vinegar. This includes the acetic and gallic acids that give the vinegar its gut-healthy pre- and probiotic features.

1 tablespoon apple cider vinegar

1 tablespoon extra-virgin olive oil

2 teaspoons honey

½ small cabbage, cut into bite-size pieces (about 4 cups)

1 Granny Smith apple, cut into thin slices

Freshly ground black pepper

1. In a large mixing bowl, mix together the vinegar, olive oil, and honey.

2. In the same bowl, add the cabbage and apples and stir to combine. Add the pepper to taste. Serve immediately.

SUBSTITUTION TIP: For a sweeter taste, swap out the apple cider vinegar for balsamic vinegar.

Per serving: Calories: 176; Total fat: 7g; Saturated fat: 1g; Cholesterol: 0mg; Sodium: 34mg; Potassium: 413mg; Magnesium: 26mg; Carbohydrates: 28g; Sugars: 20g; Fiber: 6g; Protein: 3g; Added sugar: 6g; Vitamin K: 142mcg

Fennel Salad with Avocado-Lime Dressing

SERVES 2 • PREP TIME: 10 MINUTES

LOW-CARB • LOW-FAT/LOW-CHOLESTEROL • LOW-SODIUM • VEGAN

5-INGREDIENT, 30 MINUTES OR LESS, ONE-POT

Fennel is a plant with a light, crunchy texture and a sweet, anise flavor. It's crisp, refreshing, and pairs well with this creamy avocado and citrus dressing. The lime juice, avocado, and garlic marinade may remind you of ceviche. This salad can be consumed immediately, but if you want a softer texture, let it sit for 15 to 30 minutes.

½ avocado, mashed

Juice of 3 small limes

2 medium garlic cloves, minced

1 teaspoon freshly ground black pepper

2 medium fennel bulbs, very thinly sliced

In a large mixing bowl, combine the avocado, lime juice, garlic, and pepper. Add the fennel and mix well. Serve immediately.

FLAVOR TIP: To get a more licorice-like flavor, top the salad with 2 teaspoons of the fennel's feathery leaves.

Per serving: Calories: 167; Total fat: 6g; Saturated fat: 1g; Cholesterol: 0mg; Sodium: 127mg; Potassium: 1271mg; Magnesium: 58mg; Carbohydrates: 32g; Sugars: 11g; Fiber: 13g; Protein: 5g; Added sugar: 0g; Vitamin K: 293mcg

Arugula, Pumpkin Seed, and Carrot Salad

SERVES 2 • PREP TIME: 10 MINUTES • COOK TIME: 15 MINUTES

LOW-CARB • LOW-FAT/LOW-CHOLESTEROL • LOW-SODIUM • VEGETARIAN

5-INGREDIENT, 30 MINUTES OR LESS

Arugula, also called rucola, salad rocket, or Italian cress, is a crunchy, peppery green belonging to the cruciferous family. This vibrant salad has roasted carrots that taste lightly sweet and toasted pumpkin seeds that offer a satisfying crunch. The honey-thyme drizzle on the carrots and seeds is spread throughout the salad with a light olive oil dressing.

½ teaspoon thyme

1 teaspoon honey

1 teaspoon avocado oil

2 large carrots, cut into thin coins

3 tablespoons unsalted pumpkin seeds

4 cups arugula

2 teaspoons extra-virgin olive oil

Freshly ground black pepper

1. Preheat the oven to 400°F. Line a baking sheet with parchment paper.

2. In a medium mixing bowl, mix the thyme, honey, and avocado oil. Add the carrots and pumpkin seeds to the bowl and toss to coat with the mixture. Transfer them to the prepared baking sheet and roast in the oven for 15 minutes, until the carrots are fork-tender.

3. Divide the arugula and carrot-and-seed mixture into two bowls for serving. Drizzle with the olive oil and add pepper to taste.

MAKE IT EASIER TIP: To shave 10 minutes from this recipe, consider using 1 cup of shredded matchstick carrots to the pumpkin seed and spice mixture and sautéing it all with 1 teaspoon of avocado oil for 3 minutes.

Per serving: Calories: 176; Total fat: 12g; Saturated fat: 2g; Cholesterol: 0mg; Sodium: 64mg; Potassium: 498mg; Magnesium: 109mg; Carbohydrates: 14g; Sugars: 7g; Fiber: 4g; Protein: 6g; Added sugar: 3g; Vitamin K: 56mcg

Kale Caesar with Toasted Walnuts and Cashew Cream Dressing

SERVES 2 • PREP TIME: 5 MINUTES • COOK TIME: 5 MINUTES
LOW-CARB • LOW-FAT/LOW-CHOLESTEROL • LOW-SODIUM • VEGAN

5-INGREDIENT, 30 MINUTES OR LESS

This kale salad is dressed with a creamy and delicious cashew sauce and crunchy cinnamon-roasted walnuts. There are about 10 different types of kale, and the easiest to find are curly kale, Lacinato (aka dinosaur kale), and red Russian kale. Any of these varieties provide the same nutritional benefits; they just differ in texture. If you want a softer salad, aim for Lacinato or baby kale. If you want the leaves to be a bit more tender, try the curly kale and just let it sit for a few minutes to slightly soften for palatability. I personally like to eat this salad with baby kale or Lacinato kale for a medium-textured salad.

2 tablespoons walnuts

⅛ teaspoon ground cinnamon

4 tablespoons Cashew Cream Dressing (page 164)

4 cups fresh kale

1. Preheat the oven to 425°F. Line a baking sheet with parchment paper. Mix the walnuts and cinnamon on the baking sheet and bake for 5 minutes until the walnuts are lightly golden.

2. Combine the toasted walnuts and cinnamon, the dressing, and kale in a large mixing bowl. To serve, divide the salad into two bowls.

MAKE IT EASIER TIP: Batch-cook the Cashew Cream Dressing and toasted walnuts ahead of time; you are ready to eat, mix and serve.

Per serving: Calories: 269; Total fat: 20g; Saturated fat: 3g; Cholesterol: 0mg; Sodium: 39mg; Potassium: 546mg; Magnesium: 138mg; Carbohydrates: 17g; Sugars: 3g; Fiber: 5g; Protein: 12g; Added sugar: 0g; Vitamin K: 164mcg

Balsamic-Roasted Bell Pepper and Spinach Salad

SERVES 2 • PREP TIME: 5 MINUTES • COOK TIME: 10 MINUTES

LOW-CARB • LOW-FAT/LOW-CHOLESTEROL • LOW-SODIUM • VEGAN

5-INGREDIENT, 30 MINUTES OR LESS

Balsamic vinegar–blistered onions and red bell peppers are paired with a Dijon mustard and olive oil dressing over a bed of spinach to create this delicious salad. The balsamic vinegar has a complex sweet-tart taste and may halt plaque formation in the arteries, reduce LDL cholesterol levels, and aid in digestion. When the balsamic vinegar is broiled, its sweetness shines through and helps caramelize the onions and peppers to make a crispy addition to the salad. Top this salad with a lean protein for a healthy, light meal.

1 medium red onion, cut into half-moons and separated

1 large red bell pepper, cut into strips

1 tablespoon balsamic vinegar

1 teaspoon whole grain Dijon mustard

1 tablespoon extra-virgin olive oil

¼ teaspoon freshly ground black pepper

4 cups fresh baby spinach

1. Set an oven rack 6 inches beneath the broiler and preheat to high. Line a baking sheet with parchment paper.

2. Place the onions and bell pepper onto the prepared baking sheet and coat thoroughly with vinegar. Spread them on the sheet. Broil for 10 minutes until crispy. The edges should be slightly browned.

3. In the meantime, in a small mixing bowl combine the mustard, olive oil, and black pepper.

4. On a large plate, place a bed of spinach, top with the onion-and-pepper mixture, and drizzle with the dressing. Serve immediately.

SUBSTITUTION TIP: For a more peppery bite, swap the spinach for watercress or combine the two. Of the 12 different cruciferous vegetables studied, watercress has one of the top 3 highest antioxidant counts.

Per serving: Calories: 127; Total fat: 7g; Saturated fat: 1g; Cholesterol: 0mg; Sodium: 115mg; Potassium: 606mg; Magnesium: 65mg; Carbohydrates: 14g; Sugars: 7g; Fiber: 4g; Protein: 3g; Added sugar: 0g; Vitamin K: 298mcg

Quinoa, Edamame, and Carrot Salad with Ginger-Sesame Dressing

SERVES 2 • PREP TIME: 10 MINUTES • COOK TIME: 15 MINUTES

LOW-FAT/LOW-CHOLESTEROL • LOW-SODIUM • VEGAN

5-INGREDIENT, 30 MINUTES OR LESS

Edamame are whole, young green soybeans that are mildly grassy in flavor. They have about five times the folate—a very important cardiovascular nutrient—of mature soybeans. Edamame's flavors pair well with fluffy quinoa, crunchy cabbage, and carrot slaw, and combine seamlessly with the spicy, toasty notes of the ginger-sesame dressing.

½ cup quinoa

1 cup water

1 cup edamame, fully cooked and shelled

2 tablespoons Ginger-Sesame Dressing (page 166)

1 cup shredded carrots

2 cups shredded cabbage

1. In a small pot, bring the quinoa and water to a boil. Lower the heat to low, cover, and simmer for 8 minutes.

2. Add the edamame to the pot and cook for an additional 4 minutes, until the water in the quinoa pot has been absorbed and the edamame is tender.

3. In a medium bowl, combine the quinoa and edamame with the dressing, shredded carrots, and shredded cabbage and serve.

MAKE IT EASIER TIP: There are three ways to make this easier: Batch-cook the quinoa, thaw cooked and shelled edamame overnight in the refrigerator, and buy pre-packaged slaw. All you'll need to do is assemble.

Per serving: Calories: 231; Total fat: 7g; Saturated fat: 1g; Cholesterol: 0mg; Sodium: 69mg; Potassium: 522mg; Magnesium: 94mg; Carbohydrates: 47g; Sugars: 9g; Fiber: 11g; Protein: 18g; Added sugar: 0g; Vitamin K: 62mcg

Whole Wheat Couscous Tabbouleh with Pomegranate Seeds

SERVES 2 • PREP TIME: 10 MINUTES

LOW-CARB • LOW-FAT/LOW-CHOLESTEROL • LOW-SODIUM • VEGAN

5-INGREDIENT, 30 MINUTES OR LESS, ONE-POT

This tabbouleh pairs whole wheat couscous with refreshing mint and parsley, plus a crunch from the beautiful red pomegranate seeds. Lightly seasoned with lemon juice and olive oil, all the bright flavors shine. Pomegranate seeds help decrease stiffness in the arteries, promoting optimal blood flow and vascular health. This salad easily accompanies any dish as a cooling, beautifully flavored, and textured addition.

¼ cup water

¼ cup whole wheat couscous

3 cups chopped fresh parsley (about half a bunch)

¼ cup chopped fresh mint

2 tablespoons freshly squeezed lemon juice

1 tablespoon extra-virgin olive oil

¼ teaspoon freshly ground black pepper

⅓ cup pomegranate seeds

1. In a small saucepan, bring the water to a boil. Remove the pot from heat, add the couscous, and stir. Cover for 5 minutes and then fluff with a fork.

2. In a large serving bowl, combine the couscous, parsley, mint, lemon juice, olive oil, pepper, and pomegranate seeds. Mix well and serve. The tabbouleh can also be stored in an airtight container in the refrigerator for up to 3 days.

SUBSTITUTION TIP: If pomegranate seeds are not readily available, you dislike or do not eat them, or you are in a rush and do not like to deseed pomegranates, add in quartered raspberries instead.

Per serving: Calories: 199; Total fat: 8g; Saturated fat: 1g; Cholesterol: 0mg; Sodium: 72mg; Potassium: 639mg; Magnesium: 52mg; Carbohydrates: 28g; Sugars: 6g; Fiber: 6g; Protein: 6g; Added sugar: 0g; Vitamin K: 1487mcg

Mediterranean Cucumber, Tomato, and Kalamata Olive Salad

SERVES 2 • PREP TIME: 10 MINUTES

LOW-CARB • LOW-FAT/LOW-CHOLESTEROL • LOW-SODIUM • VEGAN

5-INGREDIENT, 30 MINUTES OR LESS, ONE-POT

This lettuce-less salad is filled with crunchy cucumbers, vibrant tomatoes, aromatic red onions, and zesty lemon juice and is brought together by delicious Kalamata olives. Kalamata olives are native to southern Greece and come from trees with large leaves that take in the sunshine; the olives are handpicked to avoid bruising. Fermentation in red wine vinegar gives them their dark purple color and dense, tangy flavor. Kalamata olives are high in monounsaturated fat, a heart-healthy anti-inflammatory fat that may help reduce LDL cholesterol.

1 medium English cucumber, quartered

½ cup cherry tomatoes, halved

½ red onion, diced

1 teaspoon extra-virgin olive oil

1½ tablespoons lemon juice

¼ cup low-sodium Kalamata olives, drained and quartered (about 8)

¼ teaspoon freshly ground black pepper

In a large mixing bowl, combine the cucumber, cherry tomatoes, onion, olive oil, lemon juice, olives, and pepper. Mix well and serve. The salad can be stored in an airtight container in the refrigerator for up to 2 days.

FLAVOR TIP: Add in Roasted Cannellini Bean "Chips" (page 152) for an extra-crunchy bite.

Per serving: Calories: 96; Total fat: 7g; Saturated fat: 1g; Cholesterol: 0mg; Sodium: 222mg; Potassium: 387mg; Magnesium: 10mg; Carbohydrates: 8g; Sugars: 4g; Fiber: 3g; Protein: 3g; Added sugar: 0g; Vitamin K: 12mcg

Roasted Summer Squash Farro Salad

SERVES 2 • PREP TIME: 10 MINUTES • COOK TIME: 20 MINUTES

LOW-CARB • LOW-FAT/LOW-CHOLESTEROL • LOW-SODIUM • VEGAN

5-INGREDIENT, 30 MINUTES OR LESS

Farro is a whole grain that has a complex, sweet, and nutty taste with a lighter texture than brown rice. Farro is rich in vitamin B_3, magnesium, and zinc. This recipe combines farro with basil, garlic, roasted yellow and green squash, and Arugula-Basil Pesto (page 161) to create a sweet-and-savory flavor profile. This whole grain–based salad can also accompany a protein dish as a satisfying and nutritious side.

1 cup water

¼ cup farro

1 medium yellow squash, cut into ½-inch-thick pieces

1 medium green zucchini, cut into ½-inch-thick pieces

1 teaspoon dried basil

½ teaspoon freshly ground black pepper

2 tablespoons Arugula-Basil Pesto (page 161)

1. Preheat the oven to 450°F. Line a baking sheet with parchment paper.

2. In a small saucepan, bring the water to a boil and add the farro. Reduce the heat, cover, and bring to a simmer for 20 minutes. Once the water has soaked into the farro, fluff it with a fork.

3. In the meantime, place the squash, zucchini, basil, and pepper on the baking sheet and coat with the spice mixture. Bake for 10 minutes, then flip and stir the pieces and bake for an additional 5 minutes.

4. In a medium mixing bowl, combine the farro, vegetables, and pesto. Serve immediately or chilled. The salad can be stored in an airtight container in the refrigerator for up to 4 days.

MAKE IT EASIER TIP: Consider batch-cooking the farro ahead of time or look for 10-minute farro in supermarkets. This variety is parboiled before packaging, which cuts your cooking time in half.

Per serving: Calories: 225; Total fat: 11g; Saturated fat: 1g; Cholesterol: 0mg; Sodium: 11mg; Potassium: 443mg; Magnesium: 71mg; Carbohydrates: 28g; Sugars: 5g; Fiber: 7g; Protein: 7g; Added sugar: 0g; Vitamin K: 34mcg

Tempeh Taco Salad with Chile-Lime Glaze

SERVES 2 • PREP TIME: 5 MINUTES • COOK TIME: 5 MINUTES

LOW-CARB • LOW-FAT/LOW-CHOLESTEROL • LOW-SODIUM • VEGAN

30 MINUTES OR LESS, ONE-POT

Tempeh is fermented soybeans that have an earthy, savory flavor profile and a chewy texture that softens when cooked. Tempeh is rich in protein, magnesium, iron, and prebiotics. In this salad, tempeh is crumbled with a fork to resemble taco meat and marinated in a barbeque sauce that imparts a smoky flavor. It is then added to a fresh salad of romaine lettuce, cucumbers, tomatoes, and creamy avocado with a drizzle of a subtly spicy chile-lime glaze for a flavorful, well-balanced dish.

1 teaspoon avocado oil

¼ red onion, diced (about ¼ cup diced)

1 garlic clove, minced

½ bar of tempeh (4 ounces), crumbled with a fork

2 teaspoons tomato paste, double-concentrated

¼ cup water

¼ teaspoon Barbeque Seasoning Rub Blend (page 158)

1 head romaine lettuce, chopped

1 cup tomatoes, diced

1 medium cucumber, quartered

¼ avocado, sliced

2 tablespoons Chile-Lime Glaze (page 160)

1. In a medium pan, heat the oil over medium-low heat and add the onion and garlic. Sauté for about 1 minute, until the onion becomes translucent.

2. Add the tempeh, tomato paste, water, and barbeque seasoning and stir constantly until lightly browned, about 3 minutes.

3. Divide the romaine lettuce, tomatoes, cucumber, tempeh mixture, and avocado into two serving bowls. Drizzle with the glaze. The tempeh mixture can be made 2 to 3 days in advance and kept in the refrigerator.

MAKE IT EASIER TIP: Instead of adding red onion, garlic, and tomato paste, combine the tempeh with 2 tablespoons of salsa and mix well for about 2 minutes until the flavors combine.

Per serving: Calories: 225; Total fat: 11g; Saturated fat: 1g; Cholesterol: 0mg; Sodium: 11mg; Potassium: 443mg; Magnesium: 71mg; Carbohydrates: 28g; Sugars: 5g; Fiber: 7g; Protein: 7g; Added sugar: 0g; Vitamin K: 122mcg

Cauliflower Steak with Arugula-Basil Pesto

PAGE 72

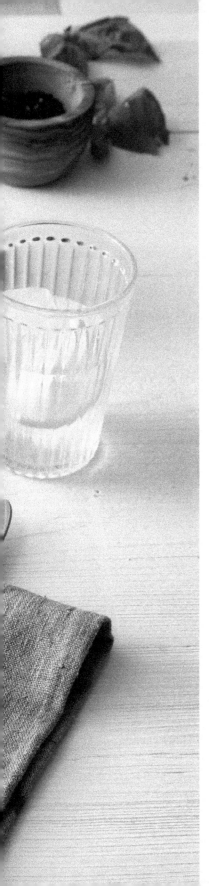

Four

SOUPS AND SIDES

Watermelon Gazpacho

SERVES 4 • PREP TIME: 10 MINUTES, PLUS 2 HOURS TO CHILL

LOW-CARB • LOW-FAT/LOW-CHOLESTEROL • LOW-SODIUM • VEGAN

5-INGREDIENT, ONE-POT

Gazpacho is a cold soup traditionally made with tomatoes, onions, cucumber, red wine vinegar, and olive oil. This version uses watermelon to bump up the bioavailable content of lycopene, a potent carotenoid that reduces inflammation and oxidative stress, especially after a high-fat meal. The flavors of watermelon marinate with cucumbers, basil, red bell peppers, and lime juice for 2 hours in the refrigerator for a refreshing, hydrating, and texturally pleasant cold soup.

5 cups seedless watermelon, cut into 1-inch cubed (about 1 small, seedless watermelon)

1 small cucumber, skin removed and quartered

¼ cup fresh basil

1 medium red bell pepper, seeded and diced into ½-inch pieces

3 tablespoons fresh lime juice

1. Put the watermelon, cucumber, basil, bell pepper, and lime juice into a blender. Blend for about 15 to 20 seconds or pulse about five times, until the soup reaches the desired consistency. It should not be pureed.

2. Refrigerate for at least 2 hours for flavors to develop, then serve. The gazpacho may be stored in the refrigerator for up to 1 week.

SUBSTITUTION TIP: Swap out the watermelon base for about 4 large tomatoes, the red bell peppers for a red onion, and the lime juice for red wine vinegar for a more classic gazpacho.

Per serving: Calories: 52; Total fat: <1g; Saturated fat: <1g; Cholesterol: 0mg; Sodium: 4mg; Potassium: 1mg; Magnesium: 22mg; Carbohydrates: 13g; Sugars: 10g; Fiber: 2g; Protein: 1g; Added sugar: 0g; Vitamin K: 11mcg

Split Pea Soup

SERVES 4 • PREP TIME: 10 MINUTES • COOK TIME: 40 MINUTES

LOW-CARB • LOW-FAT/LOW-CHOLESTEROL • LOW-SODIUM • VEGAN

ONE-POT

Traditional split pea soup is salty and high in fat from the added ham and bones. This split pea soup gets its creamy, savory texture from the potato and zucchini. It is also cooked down to represent the appropriate mouthfeel of a comforting bowl of savory split pea soup. Split peas are high in phytosterols, soluble fiber, and isoflavones that all help decrease LDL cholesterol levels. Split peas also contain tryptophan, which may help improve sleep, an important lifestyle component to a heart-healthy diet.

1 teaspoon avocado oil

1 medium onion, chopped

2 medium carrots, diced (about 1 cup)

2 cups diced zucchini

1 small red boiling potato, diced (about 1½ cups)

1 cup dried green split peas

4 cups low-sodium vegetable broth or Homemade Vegetable Broth (page 172)

¼ teaspoon freshly ground black pepper

1. In a 5-quart pot, heat the oil over medium heat and add the onion and carrots. Cook for about 5 minutes, until the onions are translucent and the carrots are slightly browned.

2. Add the zucchini, potato, split peas, broth, and pepper. Mix well and cook on a low boil, partially covered, for about 35 minutes.

3. Using an immersion blender, pulse 3 to 4 times for desired consistency. If you don't have an immersion blender, let the soup cool for at least 10 minutes and carefully ladle it into a blender. Pulse 2 or 3 times, until the mixture is combined but remains chunky. Serve or store in the refrigerator for 3 to 4 days, or freeze in an airtight container for up to 4 months.

SUBSTITUTION TIP: Green and yellow split peas are just different varieties of the *Pisum sativum* plant and can be used interchangeably. Just take note that yellow peas have an earthier flavor, while green split peas are sweeter. You can also add ½ cup of each type of pea, which imparts a beautiful color to the soup.

Per serving: Calories: 154; Total fat: 2g; Saturated fat: <1g; Cholesterol: 0mg; Sodium: 178mg; Potassium: 589mg; Magnesium: 32mg; Carbohydrates: 29g; Sugars: 7g; Fiber: 9g; Protein: 7g; Added sugar: 0g; Vitamin K: 10mcg

Creamed Spinach

SERVES 2 • PREP TIME: 5 MINUTES • COOK TIME: 10 MINUTES

LOW-CARB • LOW-FAT/LOW-CHOLESTEROL • LOW-SODIUM • VEGAN

5-INGREDIENT, 30 MINUTES OR LESS, ONE-POT

Both fresh and cooked spinach provide heart-healthy nutrients; however, cooked spinach has an increased amount of dietary fiber, plant-based iron, calcium, and potassium. Traditional creamed spinach is high in saturated fat, while this recipe is not. This recipe uses a smooth and flavorful cashew dressing to give the spinach a velvety texture that simply melts in your mouth.

1 teaspoon avocado oil

2 garlic cloves, minced

6 cups fresh spinach

2 tablespoons Cashew Cream Dressing (page 164)

1. In a medium skillet, heat the oil over medium heat. Add the garlic and cook until it is translucent.

2. Add the spinach and stir until wilted, 1 to 2 minutes. Fold in the dressing while the skillet is still on the stovetop. Serve immediately.

SUBSTITUTION TIP: To add a sweet caramelized onion taste, swap the garlic for ½ medium onion instead.

Per serving: Calories: 148; Total fat: 10g; Saturated fat: 2g; Cholesterol: 0mg; Sodium: 80mg; Potassium: 682mg; Magnesium: 122mg; Carbohydrates: 11g; Sugars: 2g; Fiber: 3g; Protein: 7g; Added sugar: 0g; Vitamin K: 438mcg

Cannellini Bean and Swiss Chard Soup

SERVES 4 • PREP TIME: 15 MINUTES • COOK TIME: 45 MINUTES

LOW-CARB • LOW-FAT/LOW-CHOLESTEROL • LOW-SODIUM • VEGAN

5-INGREDIENT, ONE-POT

This soup's base starts with mild shallots and parsnips, the latter which have a similar taste to carrots, but with a slightly more hearty note. Parsnips are high in vitamin C, folate, and magnesium, and also contain both soluble and insoluble fiber, which help reduce cholesterol levels and keep your digestive tract active. Adding in Swiss chard and its stems imparts a sweet earthiness, while the cannellini beans add a creamy touch. This soup is light and flavorful, and easily pairable as a side dish to many main courses.

2 teaspoons avocado oil

½ cup shallots, diced

1 bunch of Swiss chard, divided (1 cup stems, diced into bite-size pieces and 6 cups leaves, chopped)

2 medium parsnips, cut into bite-size pieces (about 1 cup)

1 cup water

3 cups no-salt-added cannellini beans

4 cups low-sodium vegetable broth or Homemade Vegetable Broth (page 172)

¼ teaspoon freshly ground black pepper

1. In a 5-quart pot, heat the oil over medium heat. Add the shallots, Swiss chard stems, and parsnips and cook for about 5 minutes, until the shallots are translucent and the parsnips are lightly browned.

2. Add in the Swiss chard leaves, water, beans, broth, and pepper and mix well. Cook for 40 minutes, covered, stirring occasionally. Serve or store in the refrigerator for 3 to 4 days, or freeze in an airtight container for up to 4 months.

SUBSTITUTION TIP: To add more sweetness to the dish, replace the parsnips with carrots.

Per serving: Calories: 284; Total fat: 4g; Saturated fat: <1g; Cholesterol: 0mg; Sodium: 250mg; Potassium: 969mg; Magnesium: 173mg; Carbohydrates: 44g; Sugars: 6g; Fiber: 14g; Protein: 12g; Added sugar: 0g; Vitamin K: 564mcg

Ginger, Apple, and Butternut Squash Soup

SERVES 4 • PREP TIME: 15 MINUTES • COOK TIME: 45 MINUTES

LOW-CARB • LOW-FAT/LOW-CHOLESTEROL • LOW-SODIUM • VEGAN

5-INGREDIENT, ONE-POT

Butternut squash contains dietary fiber, vitamin C, and beta-carotene. Carotenoids have a positive effect on inflammation, blood flow, and oxidative stress. This butternut squash soup is deliciously flavored with sweetness from cooked-down Honeycrisp apples and a subtle zesty ginger finish. Choosing soymilk over traditional soup stock gives this soup a velvety texture and protein boost. If you want the soup to be a bit sweeter, add 1 teaspoon of cinnamon.

2 teaspoons avocado oil

1 medium yellow onion, diced

1 medium butternut squash, peeled, seeded, and cut into 1-inch cubes (about 6 cups)

2 inches fresh ginger, grated (about 1 tablespoon)

1½ Honeycrisp apples, peeled, cored, and cut into 1-inch cubes

3 cups unsweetened soymilk

1 cup water

1. In a 5-quart pot, heat the oil over medium-low heat. Add the onion, squash, and ginger and cook for about 15 minutes, until the squash is lightly golden.

2. Add the apples, soymilk, and water to the pot. Mix well and cook for an additional 30 minutes until the squash is soft and the soup is aromatic. There may be apple foam appearing during this time; just mix it in since it will be pureed at the end.

3. Use an immersion blender to blend to a smooth, velvety consistency, or let the soup cool for at least 10 minutes and then carefully ladle it into a blender. Blend until it's a smooth, creamy consistency. Serve or store in the refrigerator for up to 4 days, or freeze in an airtight container for up to 4 months.

SUBSTITUTION TIP: If you can't find Honeycrisp apples, substitute for crisp, sweet Gala apples instead.

Per serving: Calories: 260; Total fat: 6g; Saturated fat: 1g; Cholesterol: 0mg; Sodium: 103mg; Potassium: 1208mg; Magnesium: 122mg; Carbohydrates: 49g; Sugars: 18g; Fiber: 13g; Protein: 8g; Added sugar: 0g; Vitamin K: 7mcg

Barbeque Black Bean Soup

SERVES 4 • PREP TIME: 5 MINUTES • COOK TIME: 27 MINUTES

LOW-CARB • LOW-FAT/LOW-CHOLESTEROL • LOW-SODIUM • VEGAN

5-INGREDIENT, 30 MINUTES OR LESS, ONE-POT

Black beans are medium-size, oval-shaped beans that are sweet and soft. They get their color from anti-inflammatory anthocyanins that may be helpful in assisting with blood sugar control. This black bean soup has only five ingredients and can be made mild, medium, or hot. It starts off with a sauté of a mildly bitter green pepper and salsa (you can choose its heat). Then, black beans, broth, and barbeque seasoning are added to the pot and a spicy, savory flavor is developed within 25 minutes!

4 tablespoons low-sodium salsa

1 green bell pepper, seeded and diced

2 cups low-sodium canned black beans, drained and rinsed

½ teaspoon Barbeque Seasoning Rub Blend (page 158)

2 cups low-sodium vegetable broth or Homemade Vegetable Broth (page 172)

2 cups water

1. In a 5-quart pot over medium heat, sauté the salsa and green pepper for 2 minutes, until the ingredients are sizzling and become aromatic.

2. Add the black beans, barbeque seasoning, broth, and water and mix well. Cover and cook on medium for 25 minutes. Serve warm or store in the refrigerator for up to 4 days, or freeze in an airtight container for up to 4 months.

FLAVOR TIP: Cook for an additional 15 minutes for more flavor development. Top with cilantro for a fresh, citrus-y garnish.

Per serving: Calories: 140; Total fat: 1g; Saturated fat: <1g; Cholesterol: 0mg; Sodium: 89mg; Potassium: 411mg; Magnesium: 49mg; Carbohydrates: 26g; Sugars: 2g; Fiber: 10g; Protein: 7g; Added sugar: 0g; Vitamin K: 6mcg

Persian Noodle-and-Bean Soup

SERVES 4 • PREP TIME: 15 MINUTES • COOK TIME: 45 MINUTES
LOW-FAT/LOW-CHOLESTEROL • LOW-SODIUM • VEGAN

ONE-POT

Ashtereshteh (pronounced *ash-te-resh-teh*), a thick noodle-and-bean soup often served at Persian celebrations and in the winter, brings me back to my upbringing. The earthiness of the spinach, parsley, and cilantro combine with hearty beans and thick noodles for a healing, comforting bowl of soup. It, traditionally made with *reshteh*, a thick Persian noodle found in Middle Eastern supermarkets, and served with sautéed onions and *kashk*, a thick yogurt.

1 teaspoon avocado oil

1 (16-ounce) package
frozen spinach

1 cup leeks (stems included), cut
into bite-size pieces

2 cups chopped fresh
parsley leaves

1½ cups chopped fresh
cilantro leaves

1½ cups water

1½ cups canned low-sodium
chickpeas, drained and rinsed

1½ cups canned low-sodium
kidney beans, drained
and rinsed

¼ cup lentils

½ teaspoon ground turmeric

½ teaspoon freshly ground
black pepper

⅛ box of whole wheat spaghetti

2 tablespoons whole wheat flour,
as needed

1. In a 5-quart pot, heat the oil over medium heat. Add the spinach and leeks and sauté for 3 minutes, until the spinach is defrosted and the leeks are slightly translucent.

2. Add the parsley, cilantro, water, chickpeas, beans, lentils, turmeric, and pepper. Bring to a boil and then simmer on medium-low heat for 30 minutes.

3. Add the spaghetti. Ensure the noodles are covered by the soup's liquid. Cook for 10 minutes more.

4. If water remains, add the flour until it becomes slightly thickened. Store in the refrigerator for up to 4 days. The soup will continue to thicken when stored, so you may need to add 1 tablespoon of water before reheating.

MAKE IT EASIER TIP: Prep the leeks, parsley, and cilantro ahead of time. Pack in an airtight freezer bag so you can easily thaw them when needed.

Per serving: Calories: 338; Total fat: 5g; Saturated fat: 1g; Cholesterol: 0mg; Sodium: 116mg; Potassium: 947mg; Magnesium: 170mg; Carbohydrates: 59g; Sugars: 7g; Fiber: 16g; Protein: 20g; Added sugar: 0g; Vitamin K: 951mcg

Cauliflower Steak with Arugula-Basil Pesto

SERVES 2 • PREP TIME: 10 MINUTES • COOK TIME: 20 MINUTES

LOW-CARB • LOW-FAT/LOW-CHOLESTEROL • LOW-SODIUM • VEGAN

5-INGREDIENT, 30 MINUTES OR LESS

Cauliflower is high in vitamin C, dietary fiber, and sulforaphane. Sulforaphane enhances antioxidant activity and helps keep blood vessels and arteries healthy. In this dish, cauliflower is cut lengthwise to form an open surface that picks up the delicious flavors it is marinated in. These tender, savory, lemon-flavored cauliflower steaks are topped with a fresh and crisp pesto sauce for perfectly balanced flavor.

2 teaspoons avocado oil

1 tablespoon lemon juice

1 teaspoon garlic powder

½ head cauliflower, sliced lengthwise into 1-inch-thick "steaks"

2 tablespoons Arugula-Basil Pesto (page 161)

1. Preheat the oven to 400°F. Line a baking sheet with parchment paper.

2. In a small mixing bowl, combine the oil, lemon juice, and garlic powder. Evenly brush the dressing over each side of the cauliflower steaks. Transfer the steaks to the prepared baking sheet.

3. Roast for 10 minutes, flip, and roast for an additional 10 minutes, until the cauliflower is fork-tender and the edges are lightly browned.

4. Top the steaks with the pesto. Serve immediately.

SUBSTITUTION TIP: Swap out the Arugula-Basil Pesto for the Tahini-Garlic Dressing (page 165) for a simple update to this dish's flavor.

Per serving: Calories: 185; Total fat: 15g; Saturated fat: 2g; Cholesterol: 0mg; Sodium: 50mg; Potassium: 543mg; Magnesium: 41mg; Carbohydrates: 11g; Sugars: 3g; Fiber: 4g; Protein: 5g; Added sugar: 0g; Vitamin K: 22mcg

Chile-Lime Glazed Brussels Sprouts

SERVES 2 • PREP TIME: 10 MINUTES • COOK TIME: 25 MINUTES

LOW-CARB • LOW-FAT/LOW-CHOLESTEROL • LOW-SODIUM • VEGAN

5-INGREDIENT, ONE-POT

Brussels sprouts resemble mini cabbages, a member of their cruciferous family. They have potent antioxidant properties and are a good source of alpha-linolenic acid (ALA), a plant-based omega-3 fatty acid. Brussels sprouts are also one of the highest vegetable sources of vitamin C, which helps with optimizing blood vessel health. These crispy Brussels sprouts are coated with a touch of sweet maple syrup and a subtle spicy kick of red pepper flakes that create a balanced, flavorful side dish perfect to accompany any meal.

2 cups Brussels sprouts, cut in half

2 tablespoons of Chile-Lime Glaze (page 160)

1. Preheat the oven to 425°F. Line a baking sheet with parchment paper.

2. Coat the Brussels sprouts with the glaze. Add the sprouts to the baking sheet, cut-side down.

3. Roast for 10 minutes. Flip them once they're slightly golden and roast for another 10 to 15 minutes until they are fork-tender. Serve or store in an airtight container in the refrigerator for up to 4 days.

FLAVOR TIP: To add more heat, increase the red pepper flakes in the Chile-Lime Glaze recipe to ¼ teaspoon.

Per serving: Calories: 86; Total fat: 5g; Saturated fat: 1g; Cholesterol: 0mg; Sodium: 23mg; Potassium: 359mg; Magnesium: 22mg; Carbohydrates: 10g; Sugars: 3g; Fiber: 3g; Protein: 3g; Added sugar: 1g; Vitamin K: 219mcg

Roasted Eggplant with Tahini-Garlic Dressing

SERVES 2 • PREP TIME: 10 MINUTES • COOK TIME: 20 MINUTES
LOW-CARB • LOW-FAT/LOW-CHOLESTEROL • LOW-SODIUM • VEGAN

5-INGREDIENT, 30 MINUTES OR LESS, ONE-POT

Traditionally, eggplants are salted before they're roasted to remove their bitterness. Choosing small eggplants eliminates this step and lowers the dish's salt content. In this recipe, tahini-garlic dressing adds a creaminess to the eggplant that resembles a baba-ghanoush, a Mediterranean appetizer. For a smoother texture, blend all the ingredients and make this into a delicious dip, paired with crudité or Whole Wheat Seed Crackers (page 151).

¼ teaspoon smoked paprika

1 teaspoon avocado oil

2 small eggplants, cut into bite-size pieces

¼ cup Tahini-Garlic Dressing (page 165)

1. Preheat the oven to 425°F. Line a baking sheet with parchment paper.

2. Evenly coat the eggplant with the paprika and oil. Spread the eggplant on the prepared baking sheet.

3. Bake for 10 minutes, then flip and stir the eggplant pieces and bake for another 10 minutes, until the eggplant is fork-tender and some pieces are caramelized.

4. Add the eggplant to the dressing and toss to coat. Divide into appropriate portions and serve, or store in the refrigerator for 3 to 4 days.

FLAVOR TIP: Substitute the Tahini-Garlic Dressing for Tzatziki Dip (page 167) for a lighter, more refreshing topping.

Per serving: Calories: 264; Total fat: 15g; Saturated fat: 2g; Cholesterol: 0mg; Sodium: 70mg; Potassium: 1116mg; Magnesium: 79mg; Carbohydrates: 33g; Sugars: 16g; Fiber: 15g; Protein: 7g; Added sugar: 0g; Vitamin K: 21mcg

Lemon-Roasted Asparagus

SERVES 2 • PREP TIME: 10 MINUTES • COOK TIME: 15 MINUTES

LOW-CARB • LOW-FAT/LOW-CHOLESTEROL • LOW-SODIUM • VEGAN

5-INGREDIENT, 30 MINUTES OR LESS, ONE-POT

Asparagus is rich in folate, quercetin, and glutathione. Glutathione is often named "the mother of all antioxidants" because of its important role in maintaining reduced levels of oxidative stress within cells. In this side dish, roasted asparagus soaks up the flavors of freshly squeezed lemon juice and zest. Pair this dish with any main entrée for a bright and delicious vegetable side. I like to choose thinner asparagus stalks for a crispier taste, but choose the texture you desire; just be sure to trim the bottoms evenly.

1 bunch asparagus, trimmed 1 inch from the bottom (20 or 30 spears)

2 teaspoons avocado oil

2 teaspoons lemon zest

2 tablespoons lemon juice

2 garlic cloves, minced

½ teaspoon freshly ground black pepper

1. Preheat the oven to 425°F. Line a baking sheet with parchment paper and lay out the asparagus.

2. Mix the oil, lemon zest, lemon juice, garlic, and pepper and toss with the asparagus until well coated.

3. Bake for 12 to 15 minutes, until the asparagus is fork-tender and the tops are crispy. This dish can be stored in an airtight container for up to 5 days, but is best served warm.

FLAVOR TIP: Add one more squeeze of lemon when the asparagus comes out of the oven for another layer of fresh lemon-y taste.

Per serving: Calories: 90; Total fat: 5g; Saturated fat: 1g; Cholesterol: 0mg; Sodium: 9mg; Potassium: 443mg; Magnesium: 31mg; Carbohydrates: 10g; Sugars: 4g; Fiber: 5g; Protein: 5g; Added sugar: 0g; Vitamin K: 75mcg

Garlicky Broccoli

SERVES 2 • PREP TIME: 5 MINUTES • COOK TIME: 20 MINUTES

LOW-CARB • LOW-FAT/LOW-CHOLESTEROL • LOW-SODIUM • VEGAN

5-INGREDIENT, 30 MINUTES OR LESS, ONE-POT

This broccoli-and-garlic combo makes your blood vessels extremely happy. Broccoli is rich in sulforaphane, a sulfur-rich compound that helps reduce inflammation and prevents narrowing of the arteries. Garlic prevents platelets from clumping together to form a clot, which decreases the risk of heart attack and stroke. Caramelized, roasted garlic and flavorful garlic powder coat crispy broccoli to make a perfect side dish that can accompany just about any meal!

4 heads broccoli, cut into florets (about 2 cups)

2 teaspoons avocado oil

1 teaspoon garlic powder

3 garlic cloves, minced

¼ teaspoon freshly ground black pepper

1. Preheat the oven to 425°F. Line a baking sheet with parchment paper.

2. On the baking sheet, coat the broccoli with the oil, garlic powder, garlic, and pepper and massage well. Cook for about 20 minutes, until the broccoli is fork-tender and lightly browned. Serve warm. Store leftovers in an airtight container in the refrigerator for up to 3 days.

MAKE IT EASIER TIP: If you're in a pinch, substitute the fresh garlic cloves for 1 teaspoon of dehydrated minced garlic slices, which can be found in the spice aisle.

Per serving: Calories: 78; Total fat: 5g; Saturated fat: 1g; Cholesterol: 0mg; Sodium: 22mg; Potassium: 41mg; Magnesium: 3mg; Carbohydrates: 7g; Sugars: 1g; Fiber: 2g; Protein: 3g; Added sugar: 0g; Vitamin K: 324mcg

Garlic Mashed Sweet Potatoes

SERVES 4 • PREP TIME: 5 MINUTES • COOK TIME: 20 MINUTES

LOW-CARB • LOW-FAT/LOW-CHOLESTEROL • LOW-SODIUM • VEGAN

5-INGREDIENT, 30 MINUTES OR LESS

Traditional mashed potatoes are high in fat and salt, while this recipe isn't. This rendition uses sweet potatoes, which are high in magnesium, potassium, and beta-carotene. These nutrient-packed tubers are then combined with roasted garlic, a minty hint of thyme, and creamy oat milk. These savory flavors are blended together to create a soft, garlicky side dish that has an orange color full of potent antioxidants.

2 medium sweet potatoes, peeled and cut into 2-inch chunks

3 medium garlic cloves

1 teaspoon avocado oil

¼ cup plus 1 teaspoon unsweetened oat milk

¼ teaspoon dried thyme

¼ teaspoon freshly ground black pepper

1. Put 2 inches of water in a 5-quart pot and add a steam basket. Place the sweet potatoes in the steam basket, cover, and steam on medium heat for 10 to 12 minutes, until the sweet potatoes become fork-tender.

2. In the meantime, in a small pot over medium heat, cook the garlic and oil for 5 to 7 minutes, until the cloves are slightly browned and fork-tender.

3. Transfer the garlic and sweet potatoes into a food processor. Add the oat milk, thyme, and pepper. Blend for about 1 minute, until the potatoes are creamy but maintain a thick and chunky consistency. Serve warm or store in the refrigerator for 4 to 5 days.

SUBSTITUTION TIP: If you are looking for a sweeter mashed sweet potato dish, omit the garlic and swap out the thyme for cinnamon and the black pepper for vanilla extract.

Per serving: Calories: 76; Total fat: 2g; Saturated fat: <1g; Cholesterol: 0mg; Sodium: 43mg; Potassium: 252mg; Magnesium: 17mg; Carbohydrates: 15g; Sugars: 3g; Fiber: 2g; Protein: 1g; Added sugar: 0g; Vitamin K: 1mcg

Shiitake Mushroom "Bacon" Bits

SERVES 2 • PREP TIME: 10 MINUTES • COOK TIME: 20 MINUTES

LOW-CARB • LOW-FAT/LOW-CHOLESTEROL • LOW-SODIUM • VEGAN

5-INGREDIENT, 30 MINUTES OR LESS, ONE-POT

Shiitake mushrooms have an umami, smoky flavor that when seasoned appropriately can have a bacon-like taste. They are very high in the mineral copper, which helps bodies synthesize cholesterol properly. These shiitake mushrooms are seasoned with black pepper and coconut aminos, a low-sodium soy-sauce alternative. The mixture and high temperature cause the mushrooms to shrink and crisp up, creating a perfect topper for dishes like the Kale Caesar with Toasted Walnuts and Cashew Cream Dressing (page 54).

½ teaspoon coconut aminos

¼ teaspoon freshly ground black pepper

8 ounces shiitake mushrooms, thinly sliced (about 2 cups)

1. Preheat the oven to 400°F. Line a baking sheet with parchment paper.

2. In a large mixing bowl, mix the coconut aminos with the pepper and coat the mushrooms with the mixture. Transfer to the prepared baking sheet.

3. Bake for 20 minutes, until the mushrooms are shriveled and crispy. Serve with your favorite main dish or add on top of a salad. These can be stored in an airtight container in the refrigerator for up to 3 days; they lose their crispiness the longer they are stored.

SUBSTITUTION TIP: Any mushrooms will work for this recipe. Choose white button mushrooms for a mild taste, cremini mushrooms for an earthier taste, or portabella for a meatier taste.

Per serving: Calories: 26; Total fat: <1g; Saturated fat: <1g; Cholesterol: 0mg; Sodium: 29mg; Potassium: 220mg; Magnesium: 14mg; Carbohydrates: 5g; Sugars: 2g; Fiber: 2g; Protein: 2g; Added sugar: 0g; Vitamin K: 0mcg

Sour Dill Pickles

SERVES 4 • PREP TIME: 10 MINUTES, PLUS 4 HOURS TO CHILL • COOK TIME: 3 MINUTES

LOW-CARB • LOW-FAT/LOW-CHOLESTEROL • LOW-SODIUM • VEGAN

5-INGREDIENT

Traditional pickles are very high in salt. That is, in fact, how they become pickles. Adding salt to liquid creates a brine that allows for anerobic fermentation to take place and lactic acid to form, which is the reason why pickles taste the way they do. In this recipe, the sodium content is reduced, and the pickles are flavored with garlic, dill, and black peppercorns, which give them their traditional sour dill pickle flavor.

1 cup water

1 cup apple cider vinegar

¼ teaspoon salt

2 medium Kirby cucumbers, cut into rounds

1 heaping tablespoon chopped fresh dill

1 teaspoon black peppercorns

3 garlic cloves, cut into thin slices

1. In a small pot, bring the water, vinegar, and salt to a simmer. Remove from the heat.

2. Place the cucumbers, dill, peppercorns, and garlic in a 16-ounce canning jar and cover the pickles with the vinegar mixture.

3. Refrigerate for at least 4 hours, but ideally overnight. Store for 3 to 5 days in the refrigerator to avoid becoming too vinegary. The longer they sit, the more sour they become. If you have any leftovers, add them to a batch of homemade Tartar Sauce (page 168).

FLAVOR TIP: To make spicy garlic dill pickles, add ½ teaspoon of red pepper flakes in step 2.

Per serving: Calories: 32; Total fat: <1g; Saturated fat: 0g; Cholesterol: 0mg; Sodium: 150mg; Potassium: 213mg; Magnesium: 18mg; Carbohydrates: 5g; Sugars: 2g; Fiber: 1g; Protein: 1g; Added sugar: 0g; Vitamin K: 12mcg

**Lentil, Raisin, and Pecan
Stuffed Acorn Squash**

PAGE 90

Five

VEGAN AND VEGETARIAN MAINS

Tofu, Broccoli, and Carrot Sheet Pan

SERVES 4 • PREP TIME: 10 MINUTES • COOK TIME: 20 MINUTES

LOW-CARB • LOW-FAT/LOW-CHOLESTEROL • LOW-SODIUM • VEGAN

5-INGREDIENT, 30 MINUTES OR LESS, ONE-POT

Soy sauce is a high-sodium condiment (even the low-sodium varieties) with an umami flavor that's often paired with stir-fries, noodle dishes, and rice. This dish captures soy sauce's salty, umami flavor but uses low-sodium liquid aminos instead, making it a healthier option. Serve this dish on top of quinoa or brown rice, or pair it with the Quinoa, Edamame, and Carrot Salad with Ginger-Sesame Dressing (page 56).

1 tablespoon sesame oil

1 teaspoon liquid aminos

3 garlic cloves, minced

1 (14-ounce) package firm tofu, cut into 1-inch cubes

3 cups broccoli florets, cut into bite-size pieces

2 cups shredded carrots

1. Preheat the oven to 350°F. Line a baking sheet with parchment paper.

2. In a small mixing bowl, combine the oil, liquid aminos, and garlic until everything is incorporated.

3. Remove the water from the tofu by pressing it gently with a paper towel, until the tofu feels dry. Place the broccoli, carrots, and tofu on the baking sheet and evenly coat them with the liquid aminos mixture. Spread out the tofu and vegetables evenly in a singular layer.

4. Bake for 20 minutes or until the tofu is lightly browned and the broccoli is fork-tender. Serve warm or store in an airtight container in the refrigerator for up to 4 days.

SUBSTITUTION TIP: Swap the carrots with onion for a more savory dish or with butternut squash for a sweeter one. Feel free to vary the vegetables; just make sure they're all cut about the same size so they cook evenly.

Per serving: Calories: 191, Total fat: 11g, Saturated fat: 1g, Cholesterol: 0mg, Sodium: 80mg, Potassium: 377mg, Magnesium: 54mg, Carbohydrates: 11g, Sugars: 3g, Fiber: 5g, Protein: 16g, Added sugar: 0g, Vitamin K: 121mcg

Edamame and Carrot Tahini Falafel Balls

SERVES 4 • PREP TIME: 10 MINUTES • COOK TIME: 15 MINUTES

LOW-CARB • LOW-FAT/LOW-CHOLESTEROL • LOW-SODIUM • VEGAN

30 MINUTES OR LESS, ONE-POT

This version of a classic Middle Eastern falafel swaps deep-fried, mashed, spiced chickpeas for edamame and carrots to add a boost of folate and vitamin C. These falafel balls stay true to flavor by highlighting basil, tahini, and toasty, herbal za'atar spices. Despite being baked, this falafel has a crispy coating similar to its fried alternative. This dish is great in a whole wheat pita with hummus, cucumber, tomato, and lemon juice.

2 medium carrots, peeled and cut into 1-inch chunks

2 cups edamame (fully cooked and shelled)

½ cup old-fashioned rolled oats

⅓ cup unsalted tahini

1 teaspoon za'atar (see tip)

½ cup chopped fresh basil

¼ teaspoon freshly ground black pepper

1. Preheat the oven to 400°F. Line a baking sheet with parchment paper.

2. Put the carrots in a blender or food processor and pulse for 30 seconds until pulverized. Add the edamame, oats, tahini, za'atar, basil, and pepper and blend until combined, about 1 minute, scraping down the sides halfway through. The texture should be doughy, but sticky enough to form into balls.

3. Form the mixture into 2-ounce balls and place on the lined baking sheet. Flatten them slightly with the back of a fork so they can be easily flipped.

4. Bake for 10 minutes, then flip when lightly golden. Bake for another 5 minutes until the other side is lightly golden and crispy. Serve warm with desired toppings or store in an airtight container in the refrigerator for up to 5 days.

SUBSTITUTION TIP: If you don't have za'atar handy, add ½ teaspoon of oregano, ¼ teaspoon of thyme, ¼ teaspoon of sesame seeds, and 1 teaspoon of lemon juice instead.

Per serving: Calories: 271, Total fat: 15g, Saturated fat: 2g, Cholesterol: 0mg, Sodium: 62mg, Potassium: 235mg, Magnesium: 36mg, Carbohydrates: 23g, Sugars: 3g, Fiber: 7g, Protein: 15g, Added sugar: 0g, Vitamin K: 37mcg

Mediterranean Bowl

SERVES 2 • PREP TIME: 5 MINUTES • COOK TIME: 10 MINUTES

LOW-CARB • LOW-FAT/LOW-CHOLESTEROL • LOW-SODIUM • VEGAN

30 MINUTES OR LESS

This bowl is a fresh, light meal packed with heart-healthy nutrients that is super-satisfying. The red kidney beans are paired with parsley and lime juice for a tasty and refreshing protein. Red kidney beans are high in isoflavones, specifically genistein, which studies show may help maintain blood vessel elasticity. The dish incorporates tender cauliflower and kale, crunchy cucumbers and tomatoes, and a garlicky tahini dressing for a well-balanced and texture-friendly meal.

2 cups cauliflower florets, cut into 1-inch pieces

2 cups chopped fresh kale

1 cup kidney beans, drained and rinsed

¼ cup chopped fresh parsley

2 tablespoons lime juice

1 large cucumber, quartered

1 cup cherry tomatoes

4 tablespoons Tahini-Garlic Dressing (page 165)

1. Put 2 inches of water in a 5-quart pot and add a steam basket. Place the cauliflower and kale in the steam basket, cover, and steam over medium heat for about 10 minutes, until the vegetables become fork-tender.

2. In the meantime, in a medium mixing bowl, combine the kidney beans, parsley, and lime juice.

3. On two plates, divide the cauliflower and kale evenly, and add the kidney bean mixture, cucumbers, and cherry tomatoes. Top with 2 tablespoons of the dressing each before serving. If you are making ahead, store the bowl ingredients and dressing separately in airtight containers in the refrigerator for up to 4 days and mix before serving.

MAKE IT EASIER TIP: Without steaming the cauliflower and kale, add all the ingredients to a container overnight, specifically massaging the tahini-garlic dressing into the kale for it to soften without cooking. This makes a great to-go lunch or dinner.

Per serving: Calories: 317, Total fat: 13g, Saturated fat: 2g, Cholesterol: 0mg, Sodium: 110mg, Potassium: 1168mg, Magnesium: 85mg, Carbohydrates: 42g, Sugars: 12g, Fiber: 13g, Protein: 15g, Added sugar: 0g, Vitamin K: 273mcg

Buffalo Tofu and Cauliflower Bites

SERVES 4 • PREP TIME: 5 MINUTES • COOK TIME: 20 MINUTES

LOW-CARB • LOW-FAT/LOW-CHOLESTEROL • LOW-SODIUM • VEGAN

5-INGREDIENT, 30 MINUTES OR LESS, ONE-POT

Typical buffalo wings are deep-fried and then used with a heavy cream dressing, high in artery-clogging saturated fat, for a dip. This rendition is baked to crispy perfection with a homemade spicy-sweet barbeque sauce and a touch of sriracha for a little kick. Pair it with homemade Tartar Sauce (page 168) and fresh celery and carrots for a delicious, buffalo "wing" experience while keeping your heart in mind.

½ cup almond flour

½ cup water

Nonstick avocado oil cooking spray

1 head cauliflower, cut into 1-inch even florets

1 tablespoon low-sodium hot sauce

2 cups Barbeque Sauce (page 169), divided (if needed)

1 (16-ounce) package extra-firm tofu, patted dry and cut into 8 large chunks

1. Preheat the oven to 425°F.

2. In a small mixing bowl, combine the almond flour and water and mix well.

3. Spray a large oven-safe dish with the cooking spray (or evenly grease it with 1 teaspoon of avocado oil). Place the cauliflower in the dish and coat with the almond mixture, hot sauce, and 1 cup of barbeque sauce. Add the tofu and the remaining cup of barbeque sauce on top. If you don't have a large enough baking sheet, separate the cauliflower and tofu and coat with the sauces individually.

4. Bake for 20 minutes until the barbeque sauce darkens and any exposed cauliflower is lightly golden and fork-tender. Serve 4 ounces of tofu and about 1 cup of cauliflower each on four plates. This dish can be stored in the refrigerator in an airtight container for up to 4 days.

MAKE IT EASIER TIP: Make a double batch of the barbeque sauce and easily meal prep three dishes at once: this one, the Smoky Black Bean Sloppy Joes (page 97), and the Hawaiian Barbeque Chicken (page 127).

Per serving: Calories: 362, Total fat: 14g, Saturated fat: 2g, Cholesterol: 0mg, Sodium: 203mg, Potassium: 764mg, Magnesium: 76mg, Carbohydrates: 38g, Sugars: 16g, Fiber: 11g, Protein: 22g, Added sugar: 4g, Vitamin K: 27mcg

Roasted Eggplant and Chickpeas with Cilantro-Mint Sauce

SERVES 4 • PREP TIME: 10 MINUTES • COOK TIME: 20 MINUTES
LOW-CARB • LOW-FAT/LOW-CHOLESTEROL • LOW-SODIUM • VEGAN

30 MINUTES OR LESS, ONE-POT

Eggplants and chickpeas are roasted with smoky paprika and fresh parsley, and paired with a refreshing cilantro-mint sauce and crunchy pomegranate seeds. Paprika gets its bright red color from the carotenoid capsanthin, which helps increase artery-cleaning HDL levels. Once cooked, you can easily roll the eggplant into a sandwich with all the flavors, colors, and textures for a delicious creamy, crunchy, and crispy bite.

1 (15-ounce) can low-sodium chickpeas, drained and rinsed

⅓ cup chopped fresh parsley

½ teaspoon smoked paprika

½ teaspoon pure maple syrup

1 medium eggplant, thinly sliced lengthwise

4 tablespoons Cilantro-Mint Sauce (page 163)

½ cup pomegranate seeds

1. Preheat the oven to 400°F. Line a large baking sheet with parchment paper.

2. In a medium mixing bowl, combine the chickpeas, parsley, paprika, and maple syrup. Mix well.

3. Place the eggplant slices individually on the prepared baking sheet. Top with the chickpea mixture. Bake for 20 minutes until the eggplant and chickpeas are crispy and lightly browned.

4. Top with the sauce and pomegranate seeds. This dish is best when served immediately. It can be stored in the refrigerator for up to 3 days; reheat in the oven at 250°F for 10 to 15 minutes to maintain the crispiness of the eggplant.

SUBSTITUTION TIP: Swap the smoked paprika for hot paprika for a subtle hint of heat. If you cannot find hot paprika, combine ¼ teaspoon of smoked paprika and ¼ teaspoon of cayenne pepper.

Per serving: Calories: 174, Total fat: 3g, Saturated fat: <1g, Cholesterol: 1mg, Sodium: 22mg, Potassium: 575mg, Magnesium: 50mg, Carbohydrates: 32g, Sugars: 13g, Fiber: 10g, Protein: 9g, Added sugar: 1g, Vitamin K: 92mcg

Black Bean and Red Pepper Stuffed Zucchini

SERVES 2 • PREP TIME: 10 MINUTES • COOK TIME: 15 MINUTES

LOW-CARB • LOW-FAT/LOW-CHOLESTEROL • LOW-SODIUM • VEGETARIAN

30 MINUTES OR LESS, ONE-POT

These stuffed zucchini boats are hollowed out and then filled with soft black beans, sweet red peppers, and fresh herbs, and topped with savory mozzarella cheese before being baked to crispy perfection. The zucchini boats are soft but hold their form for a handheld bite. Zucchini is particularly high in pectin, a type of soluble fiber that helps lower LDL cholesterol.

1 cup canned low-sodium black beans, drained and rinsed

1 medium red bell pepper, diced

½ cup chopped fresh cilantro

¼ teaspoon dried oregano, plus more for sprinkling (optional)

2 large zucchini, cut in half lengthwise and seeds scooped out

2 ounces part-skim mozzarella cheese, shredded

1. Set an oven rack 6 inches below the broiler. Preheat the oven to 350°F. Line a baking sheet with parchment paper.

2. In a medium mixing bowl, combine the black beans, bell pepper, cilantro, and oregano. Add 4 tablespoons of the mixture into each scooped zucchini. Sprinkle 1 ounce of cheese evenly on top of each zucchini.

3. Bake for 10 minutes, then broil for 5 minutes more, until the cheese is crispy on top. Portion and plate, with a sprinkle of oregano on top to taste (if using). This dish can be stored in an airtight container for up to 3 days, but is best served warm.

FLAVOR TIP: Add 1 teaspoon of no-salt-added tomato sauce or Arugula-Basil Pesto (page 161) into the scooped zucchini before the black bean mixture is added for a pizza-inspired bite.

Per serving: Calories: 278, Total fat: 7g, Saturated fat: 4g, Cholesterol: 18mg, Sodium: 223mg, Potassium: 1363mg, Magnesium: 120mg, Carbohydrates: 39g, Sugars: 12g, Fiber: 14g, Protein: 18g, Added sugar: 0g, Vitamin K: 33mcg

Mushroom, Zucchini, and Chickpea Stuffed Tomatoes

SERVES 4 • PREP TIME: 10 MINUTES • COOK TIME: 20 MINUTES

LOW-CARB • LOW-FAT/LOW-CHOLESTEROL • LOW-SODIUM • VEGAN

5-INGREDIENT, 30 MINUTES OR LESS

These stuffed tomatoes are flavorful and savory with a mixture of toasted chickpeas and lightly caramelized zucchini and mushrooms. Tomatoes are a rich source of vitamin C, folate, and potassium. Potassium is especially vital for blood pressure control and has been shown to help reduce the risk of stroke and vascular diseases. Choose firm tomatoes so that they hold their form and are easily scoopable.

4 large, firm beefsteak tomatoes

Nonstick avocado oil cooking spray

2 teaspoons avocado oil

2 garlic cloves, minced

1½ cups diced zucchini

2 cups diced mushrooms

½ teaspoon freshly ground black pepper

2 cups low-sodium chickpeas, drained and rinsed

1. Set an oven rack 6 inches below the broiler. Preheat the oven to 400°F.

2. Cut ½ to 1 inch off the top of the tomatoes, removing the stems. With a spoon, gently scoop out the pulp, stopping about 1 inch from the bottoms. Save the tomato pulp. If the tomato is too firm, you can use a knife to score the pulp and it should easily come out. Spray an oven-safe dish with cooking spray (or evenly grease with 1 teaspoon of avocado oil). Place the tomatoes in the dish and surround them with the tomato pulp.

3. In a medium skillet, heat the oil over medium heat and add the garlic. Sauté for about 1 minute until the garlic is sizzling. Add the zucchini, mushrooms, and pepper and cook on medium heat for 2 to 3 minutes until lightly browned and caramelized. Turn off the heat and mix the chickpeas into the skillet.

4. Fill each tomato with the mixture (about ¾ cup each). If there is extra mixture, place it in the dish with the pulp surrounding the tomatoes.

5. Cook in the oven for 10 minutes, then switch to broil and cook for 5 minutes more until the mixture is lightly browned and the tomato has slightly browned edges. Serve warm or store in an airtight container in the refrigerator for up to 4 days.

FLAVOR TIP: In the last 5 minutes, add ¼ cup of part-skim mozzarella or nondairy cheese on top of each tomato for a crispy cheesy finish.

Per serving: Calories: 187, Total fat: 5g, Saturated fat: 1g, Cholesterol: 0mg, Sodium: 21mg, Potassium: 801mg, Magnesium: 55mg, Carbohydrates: 29g, Sugars: 10g, Fiber: 8g, Protein: 9g, Added sugar: 0g, Vitamin K: 19mcg

Lentil, Raisin, and Pecan Stuffed Acorn Squash

SERVES 2 • PREP TIME: 5 MINUTES • COOK TIME: 40 MINUTES

LOW-FAT/LOW-CHOLESTEROL • LOW-SODIUM • VEGAN

5-INGREDIENT, ONE-POT

This stuffed acorn squash fills up your home with the smell of warm, sweet cinnamon, and is accompanied by a toasted mixture of flavorful lentils, sweet and fruity raisins, and buttery pecan pieces. This meal tastes like dessert, but is well-balanced with lean protein from the lentils, complex carbohydrates from the squash, and heart-healthy fats from the pecans to keep you satisfied and properly nourished.

1 large acorn squash

2¼ teaspoons ground cinnamon, divided

1 cup low-sodium canned, cooked lentils, drained and rinsed

¼ cup pecan pieces

¼ cup raisins

1. Preheat the oven to 400°F. Line a baking sheet with parchment paper.

2. Cut the acorn squash in half and scoop out the seeds. Sprinkle ⅛ teaspoon of cinnamon on the inside of each squash and place them flesh-side down on the baking sheet. Cook for 30 minutes until fork-tender and lightly golden brown.

3. In a medium mixing bowl, mix the lentils, pecans, raisins, and the remaining 2 teaspoons of cinnamon. Scoop evenly into the inside of each squash and bake for an additional 5 to 10 minutes, until the pecans and the top of the lentil mixture are lightly golden. Once ready, place half an acorn squash on each plate and serve. This can also be stored in an airtight container in the refrigerator for up to 3 days.

MAKE IT EASIER TIP: Reduce cooking time by cutting the acorn squash in half, placing it on a microwave-safe dish and microwaving it covered on high for about 10 to 12 minutes until fork-tender. Add the squash to the oven and continue with step 3 for a crispy finish.

Per serving: Calories: 412, Total fat: 11g, Saturated fat: 1g, Cholesterol: 0mg, Sodium: 18mg, Potassium: 1385mg, Magnesium: 134mg, Carbohydrates: 61g, Sugars: 27g, Fiber: 17g, Protein: 13g, Added sugar: 0g, Vitamin K: 3mcg

Chickpea and Spinach Saag

SERVES 4 • PREP TIME: 5 MINUTES • COOK TIME: 8 MINUTES

LOW-CARB • LOW-FAT/LOW-CHOLESTEROL • LOW-SODIUM • VEGAN

5-INGREDIENT, 30 MINUTES OR LESS, ONE-POT

Saag means "spinach or other leafy greens" in Punjabi. It's typically made with mustard greens. This version uses spinach, one of the highest sources of quercetin, an antioxidant that may improve blood vessel health, decrease blood pressure, and increase nitric oxide production, allowing for better blood flow. Toasted chickpeas flavored with caramelized garlic and a mixture of sweet-and-savory spices from curry powder make this recipe shine. Oat milk gives it a nice creamy texture. This pairs well with ½ cup of quinoa or brown rice to soak up the delicious juices.

2 teaspoons avocado oil

3 garlic cloves, crushed and diced

1 (16-ounce) bag frozen spinach

1 teaspoon curry powder

½ cup unsweetened oat milk

2 cups canned chickpeas, drained and rinsed

¼ teaspoon freshly ground black pepper

1. In a medium pot, heat the oil over medium heat and add the garlic. Cook for about 1 minute, until the garlic sizzles.

2. Add the spinach and curry powder and cook for 2 minutes, until the spinach defrosts.

3. Add the oat milk, chickpeas, and pepper. Cover and cook for about 5 minutes until the liquid bubbles, the chickpeas soften, and the dish becomes fragrant. Serve warm or store in an airtight container in the refrigerator for up to 4 days.

SUBSTITUTION TIP: Swap the chickpeas for cubed extra-firm tofu, which will resemble a consistency similar to a saag paneer (a cheese curd saag).

Per serving: Calories: 185, Total fat: 6g, Saturated fat: 1g, Cholesterol: 0mg, Sodium: 104mg, Potassium: 557mg, Magnesium: 109mg, Carbohydrates: 26g, Sugars: 4g, Fiber: 9g, Protein: 10g, Added sugar: 0g, Vitamin K: 476mcg

Cauliflower, Tomato, and Green Pea Curry

SERVES 4 • PREP TIME: 8 MINUTES • COOK TIME: 25 MINUTES

LOW-CARB • LOW-FAT/LOW-CHOLESTEROL • LOW-SODIUM • VEGAN

30 MINUTES OR LESS, ONE-POT

Green peas are part of the legume family, which is why they are such a great source of filling protein and fiber! They're are also high in magnesium, potassium, and calcium, three heart-healthy nutrients. This easy-to-make curry bursts with aromatic flavor from garlic, spicy ginger, vibrant curry powder, and creamy oat milk that coats the cauliflower, tomato, and green peas. The curry powder adds both savory and sweet spices to give this dish a deep, yet bright, flavor. This meal pairs well over ½ cup of brown rice to soak up the juices.

1 shallot, chopped (about ¼ cup)

2 garlic cloves, minced

1 teaspoon grated ginger

1¼ cups unsweetened oat milk

1 tablespoon plus ½ teaspoon curry powder

½ teaspoon freshly ground black pepper

1 (15-ounce) can no-salt-added diced tomatoes

2 cups frozen green peas

1 head cauliflower, cut into 2-inch florets

1. In a large pot over medium heat, cook the shallot, garlic, and ginger for about 3 minutes until translucent and fragrant.

2. Add the oat milk, curry powder, and pepper to the pot and mix. Then add the tomatoes, green peas, and cauliflower. Combine and coat the ingredients well.

3. Bring the pot to a boil, then cover and simmer on medium-low heat for 20 minutes, until the dish is fragrant and the cauliflower is tender. Serve the mixture over ½ cup of a whole grain or as is. This dish can also be stored in the refrigerator for up to 5 days, or in the freezer for up to 3 months.

FLAVOR TIP: To balance the curry's heat, add 1 tablespoon of lime juice and 1 teaspoon of lime zest.

Per serving: Calories: 159, Total fat: 3g, Saturated fat: 1g, Cholesterol: 0mg, Sodium: 188mg, Potassium: 720mg, Magnesium: 47mg, Carbohydrates: 27g, Sugars: 10g, Fiber: 9g, Protein: 9g, Added sugar: 0g, Vitamin K: 33mcg

Broiled Tofu, Pepper, and Onions with Chimichurri Sauce

SERVES 4 • PREP TIME: 10 MINUTES • COOK TIME: 20 MINUTES

LOW-CARB • LOW-FAT/LOW-CHOLESTEROL • LOW-SODIUM • VEGAN

5-INGREDIENT, 30 MINUTES OR LESS, ONE-POT

This dish features crispy tofu, assorted bell peppers, and lightly golden onions—all seasoned with a warm blend of Mediterranean spices. The red onion's sweet caramelized flavor truly brings this dish together. A tangy, fresh chimichurri sauce crowns the vegetables for a delicious and sophisticated bite.

1 large red onion, quartered

2 medium assorted bell peppers, coarsely chopped

1 (16-ounce) package organic firm tofu, cut into 8 large cubes

2 teaspoons Mediterranean Seasoning Rub Blend (page 159)

2 teaspoons avocado oil

4 tablespoons Chimichurri Sauce (page 162)

1. Set an oven rack 6 inches below the broiler and preheat the broiler to high. Line a baking sheet with parchment paper.

2. Place the onion, peppers, and tofu on the baking sheet. In a small mixing bowl, mix the spice blend and oil, then coat the onions, peppers, and tofu well.

3. Broil the tofu and vegetables for 10 minutes until the top of the tofu is golden brown. Flip the tofu and cook for another 5 to 7 minutes until the other side of the tofu and peppers are lightly browned and the onions are caramelized.

4. Plate the mixture on serving dishes into appropriate portions and top with 1 tablespoon of the sauce per plate, and serve warm. Store leftovers in an airtight container in the refrigerator for up to 4 days.

SUBSTITUTION TIP: This dish works well with a variety of sauces and vegetables. Swap the chimichurri sauce for the Cilantro-Mint Sauce (page 163) for a fresh yogurt topping or the Arugula-Basil Pesto (page 161) for an herbal flavor. You can also add or swap in some button mushrooms or cauliflower florets.

Per serving: Calories: 246, Total fat: 10g, Saturated fat: 1g, Cholesterol: 0mg, Sodium: 15mg, Potassium: 364mg, Magnesium: 17mg, Carbohydrates: 12g, Sugars: 5g, Fiber: 3g, Protein: 12g, Added sugar: 0g, Vitamin K: 93mcg

Tofu with Mushroom Cream Sauce

SERVES 4 • PREP TIME: 10 MINUTES • COOK TIME: 10 MINUTES

LOW-CARB • LOW-FAT/LOW-CHOLESTEROL • LOW-SODIUM • VEGAN

5-INGREDIENT, 30 MINUTES OR LESS, ONE-POT

Traditional cream sauces are high in saturated fat, which increases bad cholesterol and promotes arterial plaque formation. This version uses a cashew-based sauce made with nutritional yeast and oat milk, giving the dish a nutty and mildly cheesy flavor. Tofu and earthy, meaty cremini mushrooms are cooked in this creamy sauce for a delicious meal. This dish pairs well with a whole wheat or bean pasta, or on top of an undressed Kale Caesar with Toasted Walnuts and Cashew Cream Dressing (page 54).

2 teaspoons avocado oil

1 medium onion, diced (about 1 cup)

1 (10-ounce) package cremini mushrooms, thinly sliced

¼ teaspoon freshly ground black pepper

½ cup Cashew Cream Dressing (page 164)

1 (16-ounce) package organic firm tofu, quartered

2 heaping tablespoons finely chopped fresh basil

1. In a medium skillet, heat the oil over medium heat. Add the onions and cook for 1 to 2 minutes, until the onions become fragrant and translucent.

2. Add the mushrooms and pepper and cook for about 2 minutes until the mushrooms begin to wilt and sweat. Add the dressing and mix well.

3. Add the tofu and basil and stir the mushroom-cashew mixture to coat the tofu. Cover, lower the heat to low, and cook for an additional 3 minutes, until the sauce has thickened. Serve or store in an airtight container in the refrigerator for up to 4 days.

MAKE IT EASIER TIP: Batch-cook the cream sauce and then make four dishes for the week in a pinch: Kale Caesar with Toasted Walnuts and Cashew Cream Dressing (page 54), Fish Florentine (page 118), Creamed Spinach (page 66), and this one!

Per serving: Calories: 337, Total fat: 16g, Saturated fat: 2.5g, Cholesterol: 0mg, Sodium: 28mg, Potassium: 824mg, Magnesium: 111mg, Carbohydrates: 21g, Sugars: 5g, Fiber: 4g, Protein: 21g, Added sugar: 0g, Vitamin K: 19mcg

Hummus and Greens Pasta

SERVES 4 • PREP TIME: 5 MINUTES • COOK TIME: 20 MINUTES

LOW-CARB • LOW-FAT/LOW-CHOLESTEROL • LOW-SODIUM • VEGAN

5-INGREDIENT, 30 MINUTES OR LESS, ONE-POT

This anti-inflammatory dish is brought together by a creamy artichoke basil hummus and accompanied by a high-protein bean pasta. Collard greens are rich in three anti-inflammatory compounds: vitamin K, alpha-linolenic acid, and glucobrassicin. Cumin's Mediterranean flavor tames collard greens' mildly bitter and acidic one, and the flavorful hummus brings it all together.

2 teaspoons avocado oil

2 garlic cloves, minced

1 bunch collard greens, cut into ½-inch strips

¼ teaspoon cumin

¼ teaspoon freshly ground black pepper

2 cups cooked lentil pasta (about 1 cup dry)

½ cup Artichoke-Basil Hummus (page 154)

1. In a 5-quart pot, heat the oil and garlic over medium heat for about 1 minute, until the garlic is sizzling.

2. Add the collard greens and season them with cumin and pepper. Cook for 2 to 3 minutes, until the collard greens wilt.

3. Add the pasta and hummus, and stir for about 1 minute, until everything is well combined. Portion, plate, and serve. This dish can also be stored in an airtight container in the refrigerator for up to 5 days.

SUBSTITUTION TIP: Any type of greens will taste great in this dish. Use spinach if you want a softer, more delicate green, but reduce the cooking time to 1 to 2 minutes until wilted. If you are looking for a more peppery taste, try mustard greens. You can also add multiple types of greens. Just make sure you add the thicker textures first and let them cook down before adding the more delicate varieties. For a different texture, try broccoli rabe; just cut it into small pieces so that the hummus can coat it well.

Per serving: Calories: 223, Total fat: 11g, Saturated fat: 1g, Cholesterol: 0mg, Sodium: 34mg, Potassium: 393mg, Magnesium: 15mg, Carbohydrates: 29g, Sugars: 2g, Fiber: 10g, Protein: 10g, Added sugar: 0g, Vitamin K: 387mcg

Soba Noodles with Peanut Tempeh and Bok Choy

SERVES 2 • PREP TIME: 10 MINUTES • COOK TIME: 15 MINUTES

LOW-CARB • LOW-SODIUM • VEGAN

30 MINUTES OR LESS

Soba noodles are made from buckwheat and water, and sometimes with added whole wheat flour. They have a lower glycemic index than other carbohydrate-rich foods, which helps with mitigating a high blood sugar response. Soba noodles, bok choy, and tempeh are joined together by a creamy, sophisticated sauce that gains its complexity from peanuts paired with ginger, maple syrup, and garlic.

1 teaspoon pure maple syrup

1 (8-ounce) package of tempeh, crumbled

2 cups baby bok choy, stemmed

2 ounces soba noodles

1 cup water, boiling plus 4 tablespoons water, divided

1 teaspoon grated ginger, grated

1 large garlic clove, mashed and minced

3 tablespoons unsalted peanut butter

1. Preheat the oven to 400°F. Line a baking sheet with parchment paper.

2. In a large mixing bowl, toss the maple syrup with the tempeh and bok choy, then place them on the baking sheet. Roast for 8 minutes until the tempeh turns lightly golden and the bok choy centers are tender but the leaves are slightly crispy.

3. In a medium pot with 1 cup of boiling water, cook the soba noodles until al dente, about 6 minutes. Drain and then place back in the pot.

4. In a small mixing bowl, combine the ginger, garlic, peanut butter, and the remaining 4 tablespoons of water.

5. Add the peanut mixture, tempeh, and bok choy to the pot of cooked soba noodles. Cook over low heat, stirring, for about 1 minute, and then serve. Store in an airtight container in the refrigerator for up to 3 days.

Per serving: Calories: 464, Total fat: 25g, Saturated fat: 5g, Cholesterol: 0mg, Sodium: 55mg, Potassium: 956mg, Magnesium: 176mg, Carbohydrates: 38g, Sugars: 10g, Fiber: 8g, Protein: 33g, Added sugar: 2g, Vitamin K: 156mcg

Smoky Black Bean Sloppy Joes

SERVES 4 • PREP TIME: 10 MINUTES • COOK TIME: 20 MINUTES

LOW-CARB • LOW-FAT/LOW-CHOLESTEROL • LOW-SODIUM • VEGAN

30 MINUTES OR LESS

Sloppy joes are typically high in sodium thanks to their sweet and tangy dressing. This version is low in sodium and achieves the same flavor with beets and a killer homemade barbeque sauce. Tender black beans are paired with meaty mushrooms, caramelized onions, and sweet beets to add a boost of heart-healthy nutrients and create a texturally pleasing dish. My favorite way of eating this is sandwiched between a whole wheat bun and topped with sauerkraut.

2 tablespoons ground flaxseed

5 tablespoons water

1 medium beet, skinned and quartered

1 (15-ounce) can no-salt-added black beans, drained and rinsed

1½ cups baby portabella mushrooms, diced

1 medium yellow onion, chopped

1 teaspoon Barbeque Seasoning Rub Blend (page 158)

¾ cup Barbeque Sauce (page 169)

1. Preheat the oven to 425°F. Line a baking sheet with parchment paper.

2. In a small mixing bowl, combine the flaxseed and water, mix well and let sit for 5 minutes while it congeals.

3. In a blender, blend the beet for 30 seconds, until coarsely chopped into small pieces.

4. In a large mixing bowl, mix the beets with the black beans, mushrooms, onion, barbeque seasoning, and flaxseed mixture. Place the mixture on the baking sheet and bake for 20 minutes, stirring halfway through, until lightly golden.

5. Add the barbeque sauce and mix well. Dress a sandwich or lettuce wrap with the desired toppings and serve. This dish can also be stored in an airtight container in the refrigerator for 3 to 4 days.

MAKE IT EASIER TIP: You can add all the ingredients into a slow cooker and let the flavors meld together on a low setting for 4 to 8 hours. Throw it together in the morning and come home to a flavorful dinner.

Per serving: Calories: 198, Total fat: 2g, Saturated fat: <1g, Cholesterol: 0mg, Sodium: 76mg, Potassium: 595mg, Magnesium: 58mg, Carbohydrates: 36g, Sugars: 8g, Fiber: 12g, Protein: 10g, Added sugar: 2g, Vitamin K: 1mcg

Chile-Lime Tempeh Tacos with Green Apple Slaw

SERVES 2 • PREP TIME: 10 MINUTES • COOK TIME: 10 MINUTES

LOW-CARB • LOW-SODIUM • VEGAN

30 MINUTES OR LESS

Tempeh is flavored with jalapeño peppers, red pepper flakes, and a maple syrup glaze that is well balanced with a refreshing red cabbage and crisp Granny Smith apple bite to cut the heat. Tempeh is fermented soybeans that have a firm texture and, when crumbled, resembles ground beef. For less heat, swap the jalapeño pepper for a green bell pepper and the chili flakes for smoked paprika; for more heat, swap the jalapeño pepper for a serrano pepper or leave the jalapeño's seeds intact.

1 (8-ounce) package of tempeh, crumbled

1 small jalapeño pepper, diced (about ¼ cup)

2 tablespoons Chile-Lime Glaze, divided (page 160)

2 cups red cabbage slaw

1 Granny Smith apple, diced

¼ teaspoon freshly ground black pepper

4 small low-sodium whole wheat taco shells

1. Preheat the oven to 425°F. Line a baking sheet with parchment paper.

2. In a medium bowl, crumble the tempeh with your hands or a fork. Add the jalapeño pepper and 1 tablespoon of glaze to the tempeh mixture.

3. Spread the tempeh mixture onto the prepared baking sheet and bake for 10 minutes, until lightly browned.

4. In a large mixing bowl, combine the cabbage, apple, black pepper, and the remaining 1 tablespoon of glaze and mix well.

5. Divide the mixture among four small whole wheat taco shells and serve. The tempeh mixture can be stored in the refrigerator in an airtight container for up to 4 days.

Per serving: Calories: 449, Total fat: 17g, Saturated fat: 2g, Cholesterol: 0mg, Sodium: 101mg, Potassium: 775mg, Magnesium: 110mg, Carbohydrates: 44g, Sugars: 13g, Fiber: 14g, Protein: 27g, Added sugar: 1g, Vitamin K: 99mcg

Chickpea "Tuna" Salad

SERVES 4 • PREP TIME: 10 MINUTES

LOW-CARB • LOW-FAT/LOW-CHOLESTEROL • LOW-SODIUM • VEGAN

30 MINUTES OR LESS, ONE-POT

Swap out your traditional tuna salad for a simple yet flavorful chickpea "tuna" salad. By flaking the chickpeas with a fork, you can achieve a similar tuna consistency. This chickpea salad is paired with refreshing herbs such as parsley and dill, and brought together by lemon juice, tangy Dijon mustard, and maple syrup. It is also accompanied by carrots for a bright, delicious crunch. Add this chickpea salad to an open-face whole wheat sandwich or on top of the Arugula, Pumpkin Seed, and Carrot Salad (page 53).

1 (15-ounce) can chickpeas, drained and rinsed

1 cup shredded carrots

¼ cup finely chopped fresh parsley

1 heaping tablespoon fresh dill

½ teaspoon garlic powder

2 tablespoons lemon juice

1 tablespoon Dijon mustard

1 teaspoon pure maple syrup

Freshly ground black pepper

Lettuce, for topping (optional)

Tomato, for topping (optional)

In a large mixing bowl, combine the chickpeas, carrots, parsley, dill, garlic powder, lemon juice, mustard, maple syrup, and pepper. Place the mixture on top of a salad or use in a whole wheat sandwich with preferred toppings (such as lettuce and tomato, if using).

FLAVOR TIP: Add ½ cup of finely chopped jicama strips for a boost of vitamin C, soluble fiber, and prebiotics, and a sweet, crunchy texture. Jicama is also rich in nitrates, which help optimize blood flow and circulation.

Per serving: Calories: 123, Total fat: 2g, Saturated fat: <1g, Cholesterol: 0mg, Sodium: 119mg, Potassium: 224mg, Magnesium: 27mg, Carbohydrates: 21g, Sugars: 5g, Fiber: 6g, Protein: 6g, Added sugar: 1g, Vitamin K: 68mcg

Tofu-Chive Cream Cheese Sandwich

SERVES 2 • PREP TIME: 10 MINUTES

LOW-CARB • LOW-SODIUM • VEGAN

5-INGREDIENT, 30 MINUTES OR LESS, ONE-POT

Traditional cream cheese is made with heavy cream, contains mostly unhealthy fat, and lacks protein. This recipe provides you with a delicious, creamy, and savory tofu spread that is composed of lean protein and healthy fats and sandwiched between fiber-full complex carbohydrates to keep you satisfied. Enjoy the spread with tomato, spinach, and avocado on Whole Wheat Seed Crackers (page 151) or on toasted, crispy whole wheat bread.

½ cup Tofu-Chive Cream Cheese (page 170)

½ medium ripe avocado

1 medium tomato, sliced

1 cup fresh spinach leaves

4 slices low-sodium whole wheat bread, toasted

Add ¼ cup of cream cheese, ¼ of the avocado, ½ of the medium sliced tomato, and ½ cup of spinach each to two slices of toast. Top with the remaining slice of toast and enjoy.

SUBSTITUTION TIP: Swap the spinach for alfalfa sprouts or pea shoots for a refreshing crunch and a sweet, grassy flavor addition.

Per serving: Calories: 370, Total fat: 17g, Saturated fat: 3g, Cholesterol: 0mg, Sodium: 120mg, Potassium: 666mg, Magnesium: 85mg, Carbohydrates: 39g, Sugars: 5g, Fiber: 9g, Protein: 16g, Added sugar: 0g, Vitamin K: 47mcg

Veggie Pizza with Cannellini Bean Crust

SERVES 3 • PREP TIME: 5 MINUTES • COOK TIME: 15 MINUTES

LOW-CARB • LOW-FAT/LOW-CHOLESTEROL • LOW-SODIUM • VEGETARIAN

30 MINUTES OR LESS, ONE-POT

This well-balanced recipe is a true winner with everyone in my family, especially my four-year-old son, Zach! The base is made with creamy white beans, whole wheat flour, eggs, and cheesy nutritional yeast. Once baked for 10 minutes, it turns into a crispy, firm, flavorful, and easy-to-pick-up pizza. Top with a low-sodium tomato sauce, veggies, and your choice of cheese, and then bake for only 5 more minutes—making a quick, easy, and heart-healthy homemade pizza!

1½ cups no-salt-added canned cannellini beans, drained and rinsed

½ cup whole wheat flour

2 whole eggs

1 tablespoon nutritional yeast

4 tablespoons low-sodium tomato sauce

½ cup mushrooms, thinly sliced

½ cup part-skim mozzarella cheese, shredded

2 garlic cloves, minced

1 teaspoon garlic powder

1. Preheat the oven to 450°F. Line a baking sheet with parchment paper.

2. In a blender, combine the beans, flour, eggs, and nutritional yeast. Blend for about 1 minute until well combined and forms a pasty, doughy consistency.

3. Place the mixture on the prepared baking sheet and spread evenly, about 1-inch thick. The mixture will not be like typical pizza dough; it will be slightly sticky. Use a spatula to spread evenly.

4. Bake for 10 minutes, until the edges are lightly browned and start to lift off the parchment paper.

5. Remove the crust from the oven and add the tomato sauce, mushrooms, cheese, garlic, and garlic powder evenly over the pizza. Bake for an additional 5 minutes, until the cheese has melted. Cut into 8 slices and dig in.

FLAVOR TIP: Add a balsamic glaze on top of the finished pizza for a sweet, but slightly tangy addition. To make the balsamic glaze, simmer ¼ cup of balsamic vinegar with 1 teaspoon of pure maple syrup for about 5 minutes until it is thick and syrupy.

Per serving: Calories: 290, Total fat: 9g, Saturated fat: 3g, Cholesterol: 21mg, Sodium: 206mg, Potassium: 846mg, Magnesium: 156mg, Carbohydrates: 36g, Sugars: 2.8g, Fiber: 8g, Protein: 19g, Added sugar: 0g, Vitamin K: 1mcg

Carrot and Walnut Lentil Loaf

SERVES 4 • PREP TIME: 10 MINUTES • COOK TIME: 20 MINUTES
LOW-CARB • LOW-FAT/LOW-CHOLESTEROL • LOW-SODIUM • VEGAN

30 MINUTES OR LESS, ONE-POT

This lentil loaf is a hearty and savory meal that is very satisfying and texturally pleasing. Lentils are a rich source of nutrients including folate, copper, and manganese. In this dish, lentils, carrots, onions, and oats are seasoned with a flavorful Mediterranean blend and concentrated tomato paste, and then topped with a low-sodium ketchup that caramelizes and brings the whole dish together.

Nonstick avocado oil cooking spray

1 (15-ounce) can low-sodium lentils, drained and rinsed

1 cup shredded carrots

½ cup white onion, diced

¾ cup quick-cooking oats

¼ cup plus 1 tablespoon raw walnuts pieces, crushed

3 tablespoons double-concentrated tomato paste

1 tablespoon chia seeds

2½ tablespoons water

2 teaspoons Mediterranean Seasoning Rub Blend (page 159)

4 teaspoons low-sodium ketchup

1. Preheat the oven to 425°F. Spray a loaf pan with cooking spray. (If you don't have an oil spray, add ½ teaspoon avocado oil and evenly disburse it with a paper towel.)

2. In a medium mixing bowl, put the lentils, carrots, onion, oats, walnuts, tomato paste, chia seeds, water, and spice blend and combine well. Let sit for 5 minutes so the chia seeds can bind the ingredients together.

3. Put the mixture in the loaf pan and pat down so that all sides are even.

4. Add the ketchup on top of the loaf and spread thin. Bake for 20 minutes until the ketchup turns into a darker red and the edges are lightly browned. Cut into 8 slices and serve or store in the refrigerator, covered well, for up to 5 days.

FLAVOR TIP: For a more umami and meaty flavor, add 1 cup of diced portabella mushrooms.

Per serving (2 slices): Calories: 279, Total fat: 9g, Saturated fat: 1g, Cholesterol: 0mg, Sodium: 89mg, Potassium: 565mg, Magnesium: 74mg, Carbohydrates: 39g, Sugars: 6g, Fiber: 10g, Protein: 13g, Added sugar: 0g, Vitamin K: 7mcg

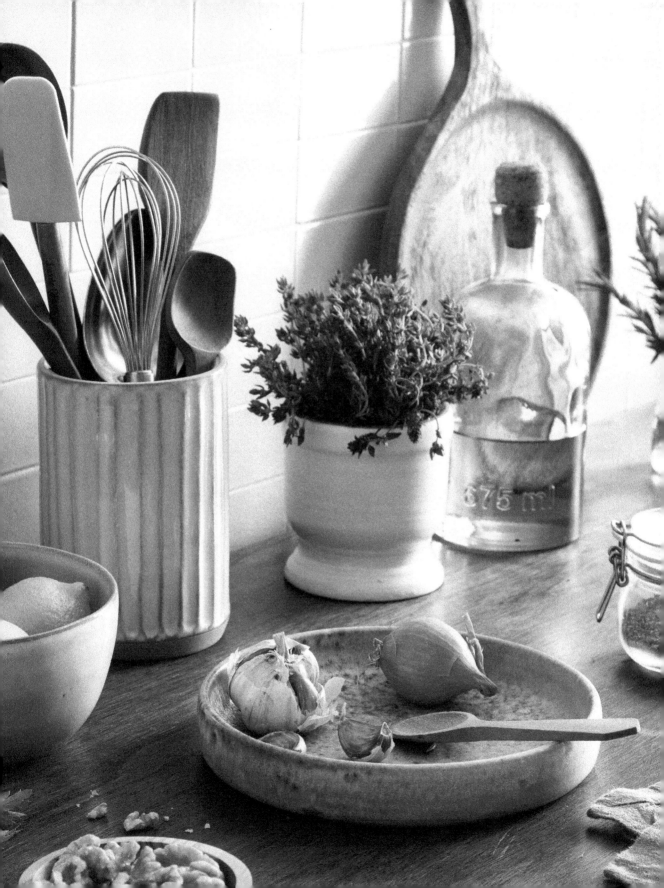

Collard Green Halibut Wraps with Cilantro-Mint Sauce

PAGE 113

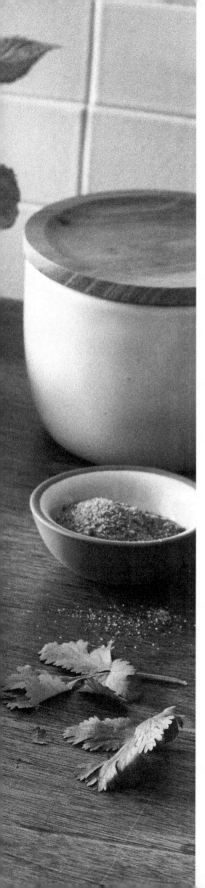

SEAFOOD MAINS

Salmon Tacos with Cabbage Slaw

SERVES 2 • PREP TIME: 10 MINUTES • COOK TIME: 15 MINUTES

LOW-CARB • LOW-FAT/LOW-CHOLESTEROL • LOW-SODIUM

30 MINUTES OR LESS, ONE-POT

Salmon has one of the highest amounts of omega-3 fatty acids, and studies show regular consumption of omega-3–rich fish halves the risk of death from heart disease compared to those who don't consume fish at all. This salmon is light and flaky, and lightly seasoned with paprika and garlic. It is paired with a fresh and peppery Arugula-Basil Pesto (page 161) and sandwiched with a nice crunchy cabbage-and-carrot slaw that is a beautiful and perfect match.

2 (4-ounce) salmon fillets

2 tablespoons lemon juice

¼ teaspoon paprika

¼ teaspoon garlic powder

4 low-sodium whole wheat mini taco shells

1 tablespoon and 1 teaspoon Arugula-Basil Pesto (page 161), divided

1 cup cabbage slaw with carrots (or ¾ cup cabbage, cut into matchsticks, and ½ cup carrots, cut into matchsticks), divided

1. Set an oven rack 6 inches below the broiler and preheat the broiler to high. Line a baking sheet with parchment paper.

2. Place the fish skin-side down on the prepared baking sheet. Add the lemon juice, paprika, and garlic powder evenly to the fillets.

3. Broil for 8 minutes, then flip and broil for another 5 minutes until the salmon is lightly browned.

4. To each taco shell, add 1 teaspoon of pesto, ¼ cup of cabbage slaw, and about 2 ounces of fish. Use a fork to separate the fish and flake onto the taco. Plate two tacos per person and serve.

MAKE IT EASIER TIP: If you don't have time to make the pesto or you don't have it handy as a batch-cooked item, just mash 1 small ripe avocado with 1 tablespoon of lime juice and use instead of the pesto sauce.

Per serving (2 mini tacos): Calories: 271, Total fat: 13g, Saturated fat: 2g, Cholesterol: 64mg, Sodium: 158mg, Potassium: 128mg, Magnesium: 14mg, Carbohydrates: 14g, Sugars: 1g, Fiber: 2g, Protein: 24g, Added sugar: 0g, Vitamin K: 19mcg

Mustard-Dill Salmon with Lemon and Asparagus

SERVES 2 • PREP TIME: 10 MINUTES • COOK TIME: 15 MINUTES
LOW-CARB • LOW-FAT/LOW-CHOLESTEROL • LOW-SODIUM

5-INGREDIENT, 30 MINUTES OR LESS, ONE-POT

Mustard is a member of the cruciferous vegetable family and has a host of anti-inflammatory, antioxidant, and heart-healthy benefits. This dish packs in the flavor and is super moist and juicy, surrounded by the flavors of fresh, sweet dill and peppery, well-textured stone-ground mustard, lemon, and roasted asparagus. Instead of stone-ground mustard, you can use 2 tablespoons of Dijon with 1 teaspoon of honey for your own honey mustard sauce.

10 asparagus spears, trimmed 1 inch from bottom

¼ teaspoon freshly ground black pepper

1 lemon, divided

2 (4-ounce) salmon fillets, skin removed

2 tablespoons stone-ground mustard

¼ cup chopped fresh dill

1. Preheat the oven to 375°F. Line a baking sheet with parchment paper.

2. Put the asparagus on the prepared baking sheet and season with pepper. Divide the asparagus into sections, five for each fish.

3. Cut the lemon in half. Reserve one half for squeezing after the fish is cooked and slice the other half into ¼-inch-thick slices.

4. Place the lemon slices in the middle of the asparagus and then place the fish on top of the lemons.

5. In a small mixing bowl, combine the mustard and dill. Divide and evenly spread half the mixture on top of each fish.

6. Cook for about 15 minutes until the fish becomes opaque and flakes easily.

7. Squeeze the lemon juice from the reserved lemon half on both fillets and enjoy.

Per serving: Calories: 171, Total fat: 5g, Saturated fat: 2g, Cholesterol: 55mg, Sodium: 76mg, Potassium: 664mg, Magnesium: 15mg, Carbohydrates: 6g, Sugars: 4g, Fiber: 3g, Protein: 24g, Added sugar: 0g, Vitamin K: 38mcg

Salmon Burgers with Homemade Yogurt Mustard Sauce

SERVES 4 • PREP TIME: 10 MINUTES • COOK TIME: 20 MINUTES

LOW-CARB • LOW-FAT/LOW-CHOLESTEROL • LOW-SODIUM

30 MINUTES OR LESS

Keeping canned salmon, spices, allium family members (onions, garlic, or shallots), and flaxseed on hand means you can make this meal at a moment's notice. These burgers are topped with a creamy, peppery yogurt and stone-ground mustard sauce. Add these burgers with dressing to a whole wheat bun, lettuce wrap, or on top of the Balsamic-Roasted Bell Pepper, and Spinach Salad (page 55). Try swapping the yogurt mustard sauce for Tartar Sauce (page 168) or Tzatziki Dip (page 167).

2 tablespoons ground flaxseed

5 tablespoons water

2 (6-ounce) cans no-salt-added salmon, in water

2 medium shallots, finely diced (about ½ cup)

1 teaspoon dried dill weed

¼ teaspoon freshly ground black pepper

½ cup fat-free plain Greek yogurt

2 heaping teaspoons stone-ground mustard

1. Preheat the oven to 400°F. Line a baking sheet with parchment paper.

2. In a small mixing bowl, combine the flaxseed with the water and let sit for 5 minutes until it congeals.

3. In a medium mixing bowl, put the salmon and separate with a fork. Add the shallots, dill, pepper, and flaxseed mixture. Mix well until you can easily form a patty.

4. Divide the mixture into fourths and create four roughly equal-size patties. Place the patties on the baking sheet. Bake for 15 minutes until lightly golden brown on top, then carefully flip and bake for an additional 5 minutes, until the other side becomes golden brown.

5. In the meantime, in a small mixing bowl, mix the yogurt and mustard. Top each salmon burger with 2 table-spoons of the yogurt dressing. Serve, or store the fish in an airtight container for up to 3 days, and add the yogurt separately when serving.

Per serving: Calories: 151, Total fat: 5g, Saturated fat: 1g, Cholesterol: 59mg, Sodium: 109mg, Potassium: 350mg, Magnesium: 31mg, Carbohydrates: 6g, Sugars: 3g, Fiber: 2g, Protein: 21g, Added sugar: 0g, Vitamin K: 0mcg

Salmon en Papillote with Sugar Snap Peas, Tomatoes, and Thyme

SERVES 2 • PREP TIME: 5 MINUTES • COOK TIME: 15 MINUTES

LOW-CARB • LOW-FAT/LOW-CHOLESTEROL • LOW-SODIUM

5-INGREDIENT, 30 MINUTES OR LESS, ONE-POT

En papillote means "enveloped in paper" in French. This recipe steams the fish in a parchment-paper envelope that marries the flavors together. The salmon is accompanied by earthy thyme, citrus-y lemon juice, sweet sugar snap peas, and a touch of black pepper. Thyme is an herb from the mint family that is high in antioxidants and may help with increasing circulation. You can swap the salmon for cod, just be sure to cook it for 8 to 10 minutes instead. *Bon appetit!*

2 (4-ounce) salmon fillets, scaled

¼ teaspoon freshly ground black pepper

8 chopped thyme sprigs, divided

3 tablespoons lemon juice

½ cup sugar snap peas

½ cup cherry tomatoes, halved

1. Preheat the oven to 400°F. Line a baking sheet with parchment paper.

2. Create two envelopes from parchment paper. To make one, take a medium-size piece of parchment paper (about 6 inches), fold it in half and make a sharp crease. Cut it into a half-moon shape with the closed section facing you.

3. Place 1 fish fillet in each envelope and top it with 4 chopped thyme sprigs, ⅛ teaspoon of pepper, and 1½ tablespoons of lemon juice. Divide the sugar snap peas and cherry tomatoes between the envelopes.

4. Close the envelopes tightly by pinching together the edges of the parchment paper.

5. Cook for 10 to 15 minutes, then carefully open the envelopes and ensure the fish is flaky. Serve with the side dish of your choice.

Per serving: Calories: 152, Total fat: 5g, Saturated fat: 2g, Cholesterol: 55mg, Sodium: 178mg, Potassium: 586mg, Magnesium: 8mg, Carbohydrates: 5g, Sugars: 4g, Fiber: 1g, Protein: 23g, Added sugar: 0g, Vitamin K: 3mcg

Pan-Seared Salmon with Chimichurri Sauce

SERVES 2 • PREP TIME: 5 MINUTES • COOK TIME: 10 MINUTES
LOW-CARB • LOW-FAT/LOW-CHOLESTEROL • LOW-SODIUM

5-INGREDIENT, 30 MINUTES OR LESS, ONE-POT

Salmon is high in B vitamins, particularly riboflavin, niacin, and B_6. Vitamin B_6 helps prevent clogged arteries by lowering homocysteine levels in the blood. Pan-searing salmon is quick, easy, and delicious. The pan-seared salmon's crispy skin is complemented by a tangy, fresh, and medium-spicy chimichurri sauce. This meal pairs well with Warm Balsamic Beet Salad with Sunflower Seeds (page 49) and Garlic Mashed Sweet Potatoes (page 77).

2 teaspoons avocado oil

2 (4-ounce) salmon fillets, skin intact but scaled

½ teaspoon Mediterranean Seasoning Rub Blend (page 159)

1 tablespoon Chimichurri Sauce (page 162)

1. In a medium skillet, heat the oil over medium heat for 3 minutes, until very hot.

2. Add the fish skin-side down to the pan. You should hear a sizzling noise or else the pan is not hot enough. Season each flesh side of the fish with ¼ teaspoon of the seasoning blend.

3. Cook for another 3 minutes until ¼ inch of the bottom of the fish is opaque and the fish is easily flipped with a spatula. If it sticks to the pan, it may need a little more time.

4. Flip and cook the flesh side for 2 to 3 minutes, until the whole fish is opaque and cooked through.

5. Plate the salmon, add ½ tablespoon of the sauce to each piece, and serve.

Per serving: Calories: 202, Total fat: 12g, Saturated fat: 2g, Cholesterol: 64mg, Sodium: 147mg, Potassium: 29mg, Magnesium: 3mg, Carbohydrates: 1g, Sugars: 0g, Fiber: <1g, Protein: 22g, Added sugar: 0g, Vitamin K: 22mcg

Mahi Mahi with Leeks, Ginger, and Baby Bok Choy

SERVES 2 • PREP TIME: 10 MINUTES • COOK TIME: 15 MINUTES

LOW-CARB • LOW-FAT/LOW-CHOLESTEROL • LOW-SODIUM

30 MINUTES OR LESS, ONE-POT

Mahi mahi is a rich source of lean protein, vitamin B$_6$, and niacin. This lean, mildly sweet fish dish is packed with flavor from the toasted aromatic sesame oil, caramelized leeks, and zesty ginger. It is paired with peppery bok choy for a delicious, one-pot union. This will pair beautifully with the Quinoa, Edamame, and Carrot Salad with Ginger-Sesame Dressing (page 56) or on top of ½ cup of tri-color quinoa.

2 teaspoons toasted sesame oil

1 whole leek (including green top), diced (about 2 cups)

1 packed tablespoon grated ginger

3 bunches baby bok choy, separated

2 (4-ounce) mahi mahi fillets, skinned

¼ teaspoon freshly ground black pepper

¼ teaspoon garlic powder

1. Heat a 5-quart pot over medium heat, pour in the sesame oil, and add the leek. Sauté until fragrant and translucent, 1 to 2 minutes.

2. Add the ginger and bok choy, stir to combine, and cover for 5 minutes, until the dish is fragrant and the bok choy is fork-tender but not soft.

3. In the pot, move the bok choy to the side and add the mahi mahi fillets so that they touch the surface of the pot. Season the fillets with the pepper and garlic powder and cook for 3 minutes, until the skin and ¼ inch from the bottom turns white.

4. Flip the mahi mahi and add the leek, ginger, and bok choy mixture on top. Cook for another 2 to 3 minutes until the mahi mahi is cooked, flaky, and tender. Serve.

FLAVOR TIP: If you want a more pungent hot-and-spicy flavor, swap the ginger for 2 teaspoons of grated horseradish root and ¼ teaspoon of honey. Horseradish is a cruciferous vegetable that is rich in fiber, vitamin C, and potassium.

Per serving: Calories: 193, Total fat: 6g, Saturated fat: 1g, Cholesterol: 80mg, Sodium: 192mg, Potassium: 908mg, Magnesium: 19mg, Carbohydrates: 8g, Sugars: 3g, Fiber: 5g, Protein: 24g, Added sugar: 0g, Vitamin K: 52mcg

Rainbow Trout Fillets with Parsley, Pecan, and Oranges

SERVES 2 • PREP TIME: 5 MINUTES • COOK TIME: 15 MINUTES
LOW-CARB • LOW-SODIUM

30 MINUTES OR LESS, ONE-POT

Rainbow trout is a member of the salmon family, having similar anti-inflammatory omega-3 fatty acid benefits and a high B-vitamin profile. Rainbow trout's flavor is a bit milder and more delicate compared to salmon. This rainbow trout dish is beautifully marinated and cooked in a blend of buttery and sweet pecans, fresh and earthy parsley, and citrus-y orange zest and juice. Pecans are very high in anti-inflammatory antioxidants and monounsaturated fats, which may reduce LDL cholesterol levels and blood pressure.

½ cup chopped fresh parsley (about ¼ bunch)

¼ cup unsalted pecans

¼ teaspoon ground cumin

¼ teaspoon freshly ground black pepper

2 teaspoons avocado oil

1 large navel orange, divided

2 (4-ounce) rainbow trout fillets, skin removed

1. Preheat the oven to 375°F. Line a baking sheet with parchment paper.

2. In a blender, pulse the parsley, pecans, cumin, pepper, and oil.

3. Zest the outside of the orange then slice the orange in half. Add the zest to the parsley-pecan mixture.

4. Cut one half of the orange into 2 slices. Put 2 orange slices on the baking sheet, overlapping each other, then place the fillet on top. Repeat with the remaining orange half and fillet.

5. Place half the parsley-pecan mixture on top of each fillet (about 1½ tablespoons each). Squeeze the other half of the orange on top.

6. Bake for 10 to 12 minutes, until the rainbow trout turns white and flaky, then serve.

Per serving: Calories: 294, Total fat: 21g, Saturated fat: 3g, Cholesterol: 56mg, Sodium: 40mg, Potassium: 266mg, Magnesium: 32mg, Carbohydrates: 11g, Sugars: 7g, Fiber: 3g, Protein: 19g, Added sugar: 0g, Vitamin K: 246mcg

Collard Green Halibut Wraps with Cilantro-Mint Sauce

SERVES 2 • PREP TIME: 15 MINUTES • COOK TIME: 15 MINUTES

LOW-CARB • LOW-FAT/LOW-CHOLESTEROL • LOW-SODIUM

5-INGREDIENT, 30 MINUTES OR LESS, ONE-POT

One serving of halibut contains more than 100 percent of your daily value of selenium. Selenium is a mineral with powerful antioxidant and anti-inflammatory properties. This dish contains a buttery, soft, and moist halibut seasoned with a medium-spicy barbeque spice blend and then paired with a cooling, refreshing cilantro-mint sauce. It is wrapped in a pocket of collard greens, where all the flavors beautifully join together.

2 (4-ounce) halibut fillets, skin on, scaled

1 teaspoon avocado oil, divided

½ teaspoon Barbeque Seasoning Rub Blend, divided (page 158)

4 collard green leaves, divided

4 tablespoons Cilantro-Mint Sauce (page 163)

1. Preheat the oven to 425°F. Line a baking sheet with parchment paper.

2. Place the halibut fillets skin-side down on the prepared baking sheet and season the tops and sides with oil and the barbeque seasoning.

3. Bake in the oven for 12 to 15 minutes, until the fish is opaque and flaky.

4. In the meantime, trim off the stems and cut out the thicker stems inside the leaves of the collard greens.

5. When the fish is done, add 1 tablespoon of the sauce and 2 to 3 ounces of halibut per collard green and wrap tightly. Place two wraps on each plate and serve.

SUBSTITUTION TIP: Swap the collard green wrap for kale or mature Swiss chard. You can also use a toasted whole wheat wrap with shredded lettuce instead of the collard greens.

Per serving (2 wraps): Calories: 182, Total fat: 6g, Saturated fat: 1g, Cholesterol: 83mg, Sodium: 114mg, Potassium: 714mg, Magnesium: 48mg, Carbohydrates: 6g, Sugars: 3g, Fiber: 2g, Protein: 28g, Added sugar: 1g, Vitamin K: 317mcg

Pistachio-Crusted Halibut

SERVES 2 • PREP TIME: 5 MINUTES • COOK TIME: 15 MINUTES

LOW-CARB • LOW-FAT/LOW-CHOLESTEROL • LOW-SODIUM

5-INGREDIENT, 30 MINUTES OR LESS, ONE-POT

Imagine an upscale chic restaurant where you're presented with halibut crowned with crunchy, bright pistachios and a fragrant sauce. You catch whiffs of Dijon mustard and hints of freshly cracked black pepper. As you bite into the fish, you notice how succulent and soft it is, and taste a complex balance of acidic vinegar and sweet maple syrup. Better yet: You can make this at home without the price tag! Pair this dish with Lemon-Roasted Asparagus (page 75).

1 tablespoon Dijon mustard

1 teaspoon pure maple syrup

1 teaspoon avocado oil

2 garlic cloves, minced

½ teaspoon freshly ground black pepper

2 (4-ounce) halibut fillets, skin on, scaled

2 tablespoons unsalted pistachios

1. Preheat the oven to 425°F. Line a baking sheet with parchment paper.

2. In a medium mixing bowl, combine the mustard, maple syrup, oil, garlic, and pepper. Coat the halibut fillets evenly with the mixture and place them on the prepared baking sheet.

3. Top each fillet with 1 tablespoon of pistachios and cook for 12 to 15 minutes, until the pistachios are lightly browned and the fish is opaque and flaky, then serve.

SUBSTITUTION TIP: You can substitute the same amount of honey for the maple syrup if you want a less sweet taste that allows the tanginess from the Dijon mustard to shine more in the dish.

Per serving: Calories: 208, Total fat: 10g, Saturated fat: 2g, Cholesterol: 82mg, Sodium: 215mg, Potassium: 629mg, Magnesium: 45mg, Carbohydrates: 6g, Sugars: 3g, Fiber: 1g, Protein: 25g, Added sugar: 2g, Vitamin K: 6mcg

Sheet Pan Tahini Cod with Broccoli

SERVES 2 • PREP TIME: 5 MINUTES • COOK TIME: 20 MINUTES

LOW-CARB • LOW-FAT/LOW-CHOLESTEROL • LOW-SODIUM

5-INGREDIENT, 30 MINUTES OR LESS, ONE-POT

This flaky, moist cod is baked with fresh parsley and lemon next to crispy broccoli. When the cod is opaque and flaky, it is removed from the oven and topped with a fresh tahini-garlic dressing that brings the dish together. This refreshing yet simple flavor profile allows the lemon slices and parsley on top of the baked cod to cut the savory flavor of the tahini. It is important to avoid overcooking the cod because a few minutes too long and it loses its moist texture and turns rubbery.

2 (4-ounce) cod fillets,
  skin removed

2 lemons, sliced

2 tablespoons chopped
  fresh parsley

2 cups broccoli florets

4 tablespoons Tahini-Garlic
  Dressing (page 165), divided

1. Preheat the oven to 400°F. Line a baking sheet with parchment paper.

2. Place the cod fillets on the prepared baking sheet and top with the lemon slices and parsley. Add the broccoli to the baking sheet and coat with 2 tablespoons of dressing.

3. Bake the cod for 10 to 12 minutes, until opaque and flaky. Leave broccoli in until it has crispy edges, about 5 minutes more.

4. To serve, divide the cod and broccoli evenly. Top the cod with the remaining 2 tablespoons of dressing and enjoy.

FLAVOR TIP: Sprinkle the cod with ¼ teaspoon of za'atar spice before and after cooking for a tangy, toasty Mediterranean flavor boost.

Per serving: Calories: 258, Total fat: 12g, Saturated fat: 2g, Cholesterol: 55mg, Sodium: 209mg, Potassium: 489mg, Magnesium: 24mg, Carbohydrates: 17g, Sugars: 4g, Fiber: 6g, Protein: 23g, Added sugar: 0g, Vitamin K: 281mcg

Pan-Roasted Cod with Pineapple-Cilantro Salsa

SERVES 2 • PREP TIME: 10 MINUTES • COOK TIME: 15 MINUTES

LOW-CARB • LOW-FAT/LOW-CHOLESTEROL • LOW-SODIUM

5-INGREDIENT, 30 MINUTES OR LESS

Flaky, moist cod is seasoned well and paired with a refreshing, sweet, and tart pineapple, cilantro, and lime salsa. The pineapple provides a tropical feel, while the cilantro and lime add a refreshing and citrus-y taste to the dish. Cilantro may act as a diuretic that can help your body remove excess sodium and water, in turn decreasing blood pressure.

2 teaspoons avocado oil

2 (4-ounce) cod fillets, skin removed

½ teaspoon Mediterranean Seasoning Rub Blend (page 159)

1 cup diced pineapple

¼ cup finely chopped fresh cilantro

2 tablespoons lime juice

1. In a medium skillet, heat the oil over medium to low heat for 3 minutes until the skillet is hot.

2. Coat the cod fillets evenly with the spice blend and place in the pot. Cook for 3 minutes, until ¼ inch of the fillet is opaque and doesn't stick to the pan. It should be easy to flip. Cook on the other side for another minute, until the cod is soft and flaky.

3. In a medium mixing bowl, combine the pineapple, cilantro, and lime juice. Plate the cod on a serving plate and divide the salsa evenly on each fillet.

MAKE IT EASIER TIP: When you're in a rush, make an easy salsa by mixing 1 cup of premade tomato salsa with 1 cup of no-sugar-added pineapple tidbits to top the cod.

Per serving: Calories: 167, Total fat: 5g, Saturated fat: 1g, Cholesterol: 55mg, Sodium: 128mg, Potassium: 401mg, Magnesium: 13mg, Carbohydrates: 13g, Sugars: 9g, Fiber: 2g, Protein: 18g, Added sugar: 0g, Vitamin K: 7mcg

Sardines Puttanesca

SERVES 2 • PREP TIME: 10 MINUTES • COOK TIME: 15 MINUTES

LOW-CARB • LOW-FAT/LOW-CHOLESTEROL • LOW-SODIUM

30 MINUTES OR LESS, ONE-POT

Sardines often get a bad reputation because of their smell and taste, but I am confident this dish will change anyone's mind. The sardines are flavored with a savory, complex, and flavorful homemade tomato sauce made with caramelized sweet garlic, fruity and slightly salty Kalamata olives, fresh and earthy parsley and oregano, and a touch of heat from red pepper flakes. Eat this by itself, with Whole Wheat Seed Crackers (page 151), or on top of a whole wheat or bean pasta.

2 teaspoons avocado oil

1 medium yellow onion, diced

2 large garlic cloves, minced

1 pound medium Roma tomatoes, cut into ½-inch pieces

7½ ounces no-salt-added canned sardines, in water

¼ cup low-sodium Kalamata olives, quartered

½ teaspoon dried oregano

½ cup fresh chopped fresh parsley

¼ teaspoon red pepper flakes

½ teaspoon freshly ground black pepper

1. In a medium skillet, heat the oil over medium-high heat. Add the onions and garlic and sauté until translucent, about 2 minutes.

2. Add the tomatoes and cover for 5 minutes, until the tomatoes have softened and their juices are exposed.

3. Drain the sardines and, in a small bowl, mash well with a fork.

4. Add the sardines, olives, oregano, parsley, red pepper flakes, and black pepper to the tomato, onion, and garlic mixture. Mix well and cook on medium-low heat, covered, for another 5 minutes. Serve on top of ½ cup of whole wheat pasta or bean pasta, or alongside Whole Wheat Seed Crackers (page 151).

SUBSTITUTION TIP: If you want a more lemon-y, salty, and nutty taste, swap the Kalamata olives for 1 tablespoon of low-sodium capers or ½ tablespoon of diced green olives.

Per serving: Calories: 278, Total fat: 15g, Saturated fat: 3g, Cholesterol: 51mg, Sodium: 241mg, Potassium: 1014mg, Magnesium: 65mg, Carbohydrates: 17g, Sugars: 9g, Fiber: 4g, Protein: 22g, Added sugar: 0g, Vitamin K: 266mcg

Fish Florentine

SERVES 2 • PREP TIME: 5 MINUTES • COOK TIME: 10 MINUTES

LOW-CARB • LOW-SODIUM

5-INGREDIENTS, 30 MINUTES OR LESS

Florentine or *à la Florentine* is used to refer to a style of cooking from the Italian region of Florence. Typically, it features protein served atop a bed of creamy spinach. This dish contains spinach, bell peppers, garlic, and a cream sauce that come together to create a delicious, well-textured, and nutty cashew concoction to top a mild, flaky rainbow trout.

2 teaspoons avocado oil, divided

2 garlic cloves, minced

1 red bell pepper, diced

1 (6-ounce) bag fresh spinach (about 4 cups)

¼ cup Cashew Cream Dressing (page 164)

2 (4-ounce) rainbow trout fillets, skinned and thoroughly patted dry

¼ teaspoon freshly ground black pepper

1. In a medium skillet, heat 1 teaspoon of oil over medium heat. Add the garlic and bell pepper and simmer for about 2 minutes, until the mixture becomes fragrant and sizzles lightly.

2. Add the spinach and stir occasionally, until wilted, about 2 minutes.

3. Remove from the heat and add the dressing.

4. In another medium skillet, heat the remaining 1 teaspoon of oil over medium heat. Heat for 2 minutes. Add the fillets and season with pepper. Cook for 2 minutes and when the middle puffs up and the spatula can easily lift the fish, flip them and cook for another 2 minutes. (Cook the fish lightly. Do not overdo it. Timing is critical.)

5. On two plates, divide the spinach mixture evenly so that it encompasses the fish fillets on top and bottom, then serve.

MAKE IT EASIER TIP: Use leftover warmed Creamed Spinach (page 66) and skip the red bell peppers. Pan-cook the rainbow trout and have a dish ready in 6 minutes.

Per serving: Calories: 402, Total fat: 26g, Saturated fat: 5g, Cholesterol: 56mg, Sodium: 97mg, Potassium: 811mg, Magnesium: 157mg, Carbohydrates: 20g, Sugars: 5g, Fiber: 5g, Protein: 27g, Added sugar: 0g, Vitamin K: 292mcg

Mediterranean Tuna Wrap

SERVES 2 • PREP TIME: 10 MINUTES

LOW-CARB • LOW-FAT/LOW-CHOLESTEROL • LOW-SODIUM

30 MINUTES OR LESS, ONE-POT

Tuna is rich in potassium, phosphorus, and iron. Your body needs adequate amounts of iron for your heart to pump oxygenated blood efficiently. Traditional tuna sandwiches are loaded with mayonnaise and salt. This Mediterranean-style tuna is light, and flavorful with finely chopped cucumbers, bell peppers, peppery stone-ground mustard, and a fresh lemony and creamy Tzatziki sauce.

7 ounces no-salt-added canned tuna, in water

1 cucumber, diced

1 orange bell pepper, diced

1 tablespoon stone-ground mustard

2 low-sodium whole wheat wraps

4 tablespoons Tzatziki Dip (page 167)

1. In a medium mixing bowl, stir the tuna, cucumber, bell pepper, and mustard until well mixed.

2. On a whole wheat wrap, add 2 tablespoons of the dip and 1 cup of the tuna mixture. Wrap tightly and dig in!

FLAVOR TIP: For a mixture that resembles the texture of a thick and creamy tuna salad, mash ½ of a ripe avocado and mix it with the tuna, cucumber, bell pepper, and mustard.

Per serving: Calories: 236, Total fat: 3g, Saturated fat: <1g, Cholesterol: 34mg, Sodium: 280mg, Potassium: 507mg, Magnesium: 47mg, Carbohydrates: 29g, Sugars: 8g, Fiber: 10g, Protein: 30g, Added sugar: 0g, Vitamin K: 14mcg

Fish and Chips with Homemade Tartar Sauce

SERVES 2 • PREP TIME: 10 MINUTES • COOK TIME: 15 MINUTES

LOW-CARB • LOW-SODIUM

30 MINUTES OR LESS

Cod is rich in selenium, phosphorus, and iodine. When following a low-sodium diet, iodine may be a nutrient that needs special attention, since the most common source is found in iodized salt. Typical fish and chips are fried in oil, which may contribute to plaque formation. This cod is coated in a nutty almond flour, seasoned with garlic, thyme, and basil and baked on high heat for a crispy fish tender. Dip it into a savory homemade tartar sauce made with yogurt, pickles, and dill, and pair it with thin and crispy zucchini chips.

1 large zucchini

2 egg whites

½ cup almond meal

1 large garlic clove, minced

1¼ teaspoon dried thyme, divided

1¼ teaspoon dried basil, divided

2 (4-ounce) cod fillets, skinned and cut into 1-inch strips

1 teaspoon avocado oil

¼ teaspoon freshly ground black pepper

4 tablespoons Tartar Sauce (page 168)

1. Preheat the oven to 425°F. Line a baking sheet with parchment paper.

2. Thinly cut the zucchini into small coins. Press the coins with paper towels to draw out excess moisture. The drier you get the coins, the crispier they'll get.

3. In a medium bowl, beat the egg whites. On a medium shallow plate, combine the almond meal, garlic, 1 teaspoon of thyme, and 1 teaspoon of basil, and mix well.

4. Coat the fish strips on both sides with the egg whites. Dredge the fish strips in the almond meal mixture and coat well.

5. Place each strip separately on the prepared baking sheet.

6. In a medium mixing bowl, combine the oil, pepper, and the remaining ¼ teaspoon of thyme and ¼ teaspoon of basil. Add the zucchini coins and toss to coat evenly. Place separately on the baking sheet.

7. Bake for 12 minutes, flipping the fish halfway through, until lightly golden on each side. The zucchini chips should have no excess oil and be crisp. The zucchini chips can be stored in a zip-top bag or an airtight container for 7 days.

FLAVOR TIP: Use 1 tablespoon and 1 teaspoon of fresh thyme instead of dried for added minty, earthy flavor and smell.

Per serving: Calories: 328, Total fat: 17g, Saturated fat: 2g, Cholesterol: 57mg, Sodium: 239mg, Potassium: 1025mg, Magnesium: 116mg, Carbohydrates: 13g, Sugars: 7g, Fiber: 5g, Protein: 32g, Added sugar: 0g, Vitamin K: 19mcg

Baked Chicken Shawarma

PAGE 129

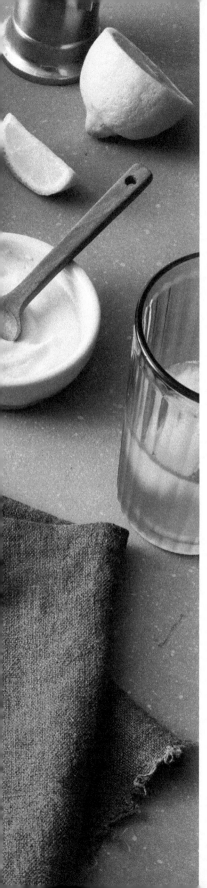

Seven

LEAN POULTRY

Tahini and Turmeric Chicken Salad

SERVES 2 • PREP TIME: 10 MINUTES • COOK TIME: 10 MINUTES

LOW-CARB • LOW-SODIUM

30 MINUTES OR LESS, ONE-POT

Traditional chicken salad uses unhealthy, heavily processed mayonnaise. This recipe replaces mayo with nutty and creamy tahini, which adds flavor and nutrients such as copper, magnesium, and zinc. The tahini dressing is paired with anti-inflammatory turmeric and coats moist, juicy chicken cubes—all balanced with crisp, refreshing Honeycrisp apples and celery. Add this mixture to an open-face sandwich, serve inside a lettuce wrap, or swap it for the kidney bean salad in the Mediterranean Bowl (page 84).

2 teaspoons avocado oil

2 large garlic cloves, minced

1 (8-ounce) chicken breast, cubed

3 tablespoons unsalted tahini

½ teaspoon ground turmeric

¼ teaspoon freshly ground black pepper

1 tablespoon lemon juice

2 tablespoons water

2 celery stalks, diced

1 Honeycrisp apple, cut into ½-inch pieces

1. In a medium skillet, heat the oil and garlic over medium heat for 2 minutes, until the garlic is sizzling and translucent.

2. Add the chicken breast and cook for 4 minutes on one side, until the chicken is ⅔ white around the bottom. Flip and cook for another 2 minutes, until the browned chicken is lightly golden and cooked through.

3. In a large mixing bowl, add the tahini, turmeric, pepper, lemon juice, and water and combine thoroughly. Add in the browned chicken breast, celery, and apples and mix well.

4. Enjoy over a lettuce wrap, salad, or on one or two slices of whole wheat bread. Store in an airtight container in the refrigerator for up to 3 days.

MAKE IT EASIER TIP: If you have Tahini-Garlic Dressing (page 165) batch-cooked, add ½ teaspoon of turmeric to it, mix well, and place it on top of the cooked, cubed chicken.

Per serving: Calories: 366, Total fat: 20g, Saturated fat: 2g, Cholesterol: 80mg, Sodium: 112mg, Potassium: 238mg, Magnesium: 29mg, Carbohydrates: 21g, Sugars: 11g, Fiber: 5g, Protein: 29g, Added sugar: 0g, Vitamin K: 7mcg

Chicken Lettuce Wrap with Peanut Dressing

SERVES 2 • PREP TIME: 10 MINUTES • COOK TIME: 5 MINUTES

LOW-CARB • LOW-SODIUM

30 MINUTES OR LESS

If you love peanut butter, you must try this dish! Smooth and creamy peanut butter is mixed with a zesty ginger and a subtle garlicky taste for a dressing perfectly suited for sautéed ground chicken. Peanut butter is a rich source of magnesium, prebiotics, and resveratrol, a potent antioxidant that has heart-healthy, anti-inflammatory properties. The butter lettuce leaves scoop up the chicken marinated in peanut butter, garlic, and ginger to make a delicious bite that just melts in your mouth.

2 teaspoons avocado oil

2 garlic cloves, minced, divided

½ cup diced shallots

8 ounces lean ground chicken or turkey breast

1 teaspoon grated ginger

3 tablespoons unsalted peanut butter

4 tablespoons water

6 large butter lettuce leaves

1. In a medium skillet, heat the oil over medium heat. Add 1 minced garlic clove and the shallots and cook for 1 to 2 minutes, until sizzling and translucent.

2. Add the ground chicken and break into pieces. Stir the ground meat until lightly golden and cooked through, about 5 minutes.

3. In a small mixing bowl, combine the ginger, remaining garlic clove, peanut butter, and water. Add to the chicken mixture on the stovetop. Cook for about 1 minute until all flavors have combined.

4. Divide the chicken mixture into the lettuce cups and serve. Alternatively, this dish can be stored in an airtight container in the refrigerator for up to 3 days.

MAKE IT EASIER TIP: Double a batch of the peanut butter sauce for the chicken lettuce wraps and for the Soba Noodles with Peanut Tempeh and Bok Choy (page 96) to decrease meal prep time and make two meals at once.

Per serving: Calories: 414, Total fat: 21g, Saturated fat: 4g, Cholesterol: 90mg, Sodium: 211mg, Potassium: 590mg, Magnesium: 65mg, Carbohydrates: 17g, Sugars: 7g, Fiber: 4g, Protein: 32g, Added sugar: 0g, Vitamin K: 47mcg

Stovetop Shredded Chicken

SERVES 2 • PREP TIME: 10 MINUTES • COOK TIME: 15 MINUTES
LOW-CARB • LOW-FAT/LOW-CHOLESTEROL • LOW-SODIUM

30 MINUTES OR LESS, ONE-POT

This stovetop shredded chicken is a hearty one-pot meal complemented by sweet onions, savory white beans, and a mild spicy kick from the barbeque seasoning. It is finished with the citrus-y flair of lime juice that balances and brings the whole dish together. Add this to a whole wheat soft-shell taco with shredded lettuce on top, or replace the tempeh crumble for this dish in the Tempeh Taco Salad with Chile-Lime Glaze (page 60).

2 (4-ounce) chicken breasts

2 cups low-sodium veggie broth or Homemade Vegetable Broth (page 172)

2 tablespoons lime juice

2 garlic cloves, minced

1 cup cannellini beans drained and rinsed

1 teaspoon Barbeque Seasoning Rub Blend (page 158)

1. In a medium pot, cook the chicken breasts and veggie broth over medium heat for 10 minutes, until the chicken is cooked through and is easily shredded.

2. In the pot, carefully shred the chicken with two forks and then add the lime juice, garlic, beans, and barbeque seasoning. Stir well and cover for another 5 minutes until all the flavors are blended together, and the beans and onions have softened. Serve on top of a salad, lettuce cup, or whole wheat soft taco shell. Alternatively, the chicken may be stored in an airtight container in the refrigerator for up to 3 days.

SUBSTITUTION TIP: Swap the low-sodium veggie broth for low-sodium chicken bone broth to give the chicken a more savory, meaty, and rich flavor. Chicken bone broth also adds a boost of calcium and magnesium, which are beneficial to your heart health.

Per serving: Calories: 301, Total fat: 6g, Saturated fat: 1g, Cholesterol: 80mg, Sodium: 193mg, Potassium: 287mg, Magnesium: 15mg, Carbohydrates: 25g, Sugars: 3g, Fiber: 8g, Protein: 34g, Added sugar: 0g, Vitamin K: 3mcg

Hawaiian Barbeque Chicken

SERVES 2 • PREP TIME: 5 MINUTES • COOK TIME: 20 MINUTES

LOW-CARB • LOW-FAT/LOW-CHOLESTEROL • LOW-SODIUM

5-INGREDIENT, 30 MINUTES OR LESS, ONE-POT

Typical barbeque chicken is loaded with saturated fat from dark meat chicken and salt from the barbeque sauce. Lean chicken breast, which is used in this dish, is three times leaner than dark meat chicken thighs. This barbeque chicken is coated with sesame seeds for a toasted sesame flavor. It also has a nice, medium spice level from the barbeque sauce that is balanced by the sweet tanginess of the caramelized pineapples and the slightly bitter crunch of green bell peppers. It pairs well with the cooling Fennel Salad with Avocado-Lime Dressing (page 52).

2 (4-ounce) chicken breasts, flattened 1-inch thick

2 teaspoons sesame seeds

1 cup diced pineapple

1 cup diced green bell peppers

1 cup Barbeque Sauce (page 169)

1. Preheat the oven to 400°F. Line a baking sheet with parchment paper.

2. Place the chicken on the prepared baking sheet and top with sesame seeds. Surround the chicken with the pineapple and green peppers. Coat the chicken with barbeque sauce and cook for 10 to 15 minutes, until the pineapple is caramelized and the chicken is cooked through. Serve with a side of your choice, or store in an airtight container in the refrigerator for up to 3 days.

FLAVOR TIP: Add 2 tablespoons of scallion tops as a garnish for a mild onion taste and a nice textural crunch.

Per serving: Calories: 327, Total fat: 6g, Saturated fat: 1g, Cholesterol: 80mg, Sodium: 206mg, Potassium: 356mg, Magnesium: 47mg, Carbohydrates: 23g, Sugars: 24g, Fiber: 7g, Protein: 31g, Added sugar: 4g, Vitamin K: 6mcg

Cilantro-Lime Chicken

SERVES 2 • PREP TIME: 5 MINUTES • COOK TIME: 10 MINUTES

LOW-CARB • LOW-FAT/LOW-CHOLESTEROL • LOW-SODIUM

5-INGREDIENT, 30 MINUTES OR LESS, ONE-POT

This light chicken is marinated with red pepper flakes, maple syrup, and cilantro for a modestly spicy yet surprisingly sweet dish. This dish is versatile and can be used in a variety of ways—you can use a whole chicken breast, slice the chicken into cubes or strips, or swap it for the tempeh in the Chile-Lime Tempeh Tacos with Green Apple Slaw (page 98) or in the Tempeh Taco Salad with Chile-Lime Glaze (page 60). It also pairs well with the Red Cabbage and Apple Salad with Apple Cider Vinegar and Honey Dressing (page 51).

2 (4-ounce) chicken breasts

2 tablespoons Chile-Lime Glaze (page 160)

¼ teaspoon garlic powder

¼ teaspoon freshly ground black pepper

2 tablespoons chopped fresh cilantro

2 tablespoons lime juice

1. In a large mixing bowl or freezer bag, marinate the chicken with the glaze, garlic powder, pepper, and cilantro for at least 10 minutes.

2. In a medium skillet over medium-low heat, cook the chicken for 5 to 7 minutes on each side, until lightly browned and cooked through. Add the lime juice over the chicken. Serve on salad or paired with a side dish of your choice. Alternatively, the chicken may be stored in an airtight container in the refrigerator for up to 3 days.

FLAVOR TIP: Marinate the chicken for 4 hours or overnight for a richer and more pronounced chile-lime and maple syrup flavor.

Per serving: Calories: 184, Total fat: 8g, Saturated fat: 1g, Cholesterol: 80mg, Sodium: 52mg, Potassium: 48mg, Magnesium: 4mg, Carbohydrates: 4g, Sugars: 2g, Fiber: <1g, Protein: 25g, Added sugar: 1g, Vitamin K: 6mcg

Baked Chicken Shawarma

SERVES 2 • PREP TIME: 5 MINUTES • COOK TIME: 15 MINUTES

LOW-CARB • LOW-FAT/LOW-CHOLESTEROL • LOW-SODIUM

5-INGREDIENT, 30 MINUTES OR LESS, ONE-POT

Shawarma is a Middle Eastern dish that, while delicious, is typically high in saturated fat and calories. This rendition uses lean chicken breast marinated in a paste-like wet rub of Mediterranean spices and lemon juice, and cooked over a bed of caramelized onions that keeps the chicken tender. Serve this warm, well-seasoned shawarma in a toasted pita pocket with a handful of arugula, Roasted Eggplant with Tahini-Garlic Dressing (page 74), and bite-size cucumbers and tomatoes.

2 tablespoons Mediterranean Seasoning Rub Blend (page 159)

4 teaspoons avocado oil

2 tablespoons lemon juice

8 ounces chicken, cut into 1-inch cubes

1 large red onion, cut into rings

1. Preheat the oven to 450°F. Line a baking sheet with parchment paper.

2. In a large mixing bowl, combine the seasoning blend, oil, and lemon juice. Add the chicken and coat well with the mixture. Let marinate for at least 5 minutes; the longer it marinates the more flavor it will have.

3. Place the onions on the prepared baking sheet, add the chicken on top, and bake for 12 to 15 minutes, until the onions are caramelized and the chicken is lightly browned. Serve with your desired toppings and enjoy. Store in an airtight container in the refrigerator for up to 3 days.

FLAVOR TIP: To add a caramelized crust and subtly sweet complement to the chicken, add 1 teaspoon of maple syrup and 1 teaspoon of cinnamon to the seasoning blend.

Per serving: Calories: 266, Total fat: 12g, Saturated fat: 2g, Cholesterol: 80mg, Sodium: 57mg, Potassium: 230mg, Magnesium: 19mg, Carbohydrates: 13g, Sugars: 4g, Fiber: 2g, Protein: 27g, Added sugar: 0g, Vitamin K: 3mcg

Lemon-Basil Chicken with Baby Bell Peppers

SERVES 2 • PREP TIME: 10 MINUTES • COOK TIME: 20 MINUTES
LOW-CARB • LOW-FAT/LOW-CHOLESTEROL • LOW-SODIUM

5-INGREDIENT, 30 MINUTES OR LESS, ONE-POT

This simple sheet pan recipe is deliciously flavored with a Mediterranean seasoning blend, lemon juice, and fresh basil. The chicken is moist and juicy, while the baby bell peppers are fork-tender for a nice crunch. You can also cook the baby bell peppers for 5 to 10 minutes longer until blistered if you like them softer. If you cannot find baby bell peppers, substitute them with 1 cup of diced regular-size bell peppers. This dish pairs well with the Roasted Summer Squash Farro Salad (page 59).

8 ounces chicken breast, cubed

4 cups baby bell peppers

¾ teaspoon Mediterranean Seasoning Rub Blend (page 159)

2 heaping tablespoons chopped fresh basil

2 tablespoons lemon juice

1 teaspoon avocado oil

1. Preheat the oven to 375°F. Line a baking sheet with parchment paper and place the chicken and bell peppers on top.

2. In a small bowl, mix the seasoning blend, basil, lemon juice, and oil. Coat all the pieces evenly with the seasoning mixture on the baking sheet.

3. Bake for 20 minutes, until the chicken is slightly golden and cooked through, and the bell peppers are fork-tender. Divide into even portions and serve. Alternatively, this dish may be stored in the refrigerator in an airtight container for up to 3 days.

SUBSTITUTION TIP: Instead of flavoring the chicken with the seasoning blend, combine 1 teaspoon of sumac and ¼ teaspoon of allspice for a more subtle sweet, citrus flavor.

Per serving: Calories: 185, Total fat: 6g, Saturated fat: 1g, Cholesterol: 80mg, Sodium: 55mg, Potassium: 234mg, Magnesium: 17mg, Carbohydrates: 8g, Sugars: 4g, Fiber: 2g, Protein: 26g, Added sugar: 0g, Vitamin K: 24mcg

Sesame and Pumpkin Seed Chicken Tenders

SERVES 2 • PREP TIME: 15 MINUTES • COOK TIME: 15 MINUTES

LOW-CARB • LOW-FAT/LOW-CHOLESTEROL • LOW-SODIUM

5-INGREDIENT, 30 MINUTES OR LESS

Chicken tenders are typically high in salt and deep-fried, adding saturated fat and trans fatty acids into your diet. These chicken tenders are made with lean, baked chicken breasts surrounded by heart-healthy polyunsaturated seeds. They obtain their crispy outer crunch from sesame seeds and crushed pumpkin seeds, while maintaining a moist and juicy interior. Tahini-Garlic Dressing (page 165) works as an excellent dip, and the tenders pair well with Cheesy Kale Chips (page 153).

2½ tablespoons unsalted raw pumpkin seeds, crushed

2 tablespoons unsalted raw sesame seeds

½ teaspoon freshly ground black pepper

1 teaspoon dried oregano

2 egg whites

8 ounces chicken breast, cut into 1-inch-thick, 2-inch-long strips

1. Preheat the oven to 400°F. Line a baking sheet with parchment paper.

2. In a medium mixing bowl, mix the pumpkin seeds, sesame seeds, pepper, and oregano. In a shallow medium bowl, pour the egg whites.

3. Dip both sides of the chicken strips into the egg mixture, and then fully coat each strip with the seed mixture. Place them on the baking sheet and cook for 10 minutes, until the seeds are lightly browned and the chicken is cooked through. Divide and serve with a side of your choice. Store in an airtight container in the refrigerator for up to 3 days.

FLAVOR TIP: Add 1 teaspoon of finely chopped fresh sage to the seed mixture for a sweet and slightly bitter flavor enhancement.

Per serving: Calories: 259, Total fat: 13g, Saturated fat: 2g, Cholesterol: 80mg, Sodium: 75mg, Potassium: 165mg, Magnesium: 88mg, Carbohydrates: 3g, Sugars: <1g, Fiber: 2g, Protein: 33g, Added sugar: 0g, Vitamin K: 4mcg

Chicken Fajitas with Red and Yellow Bell Peppers

SERVES 2 • PREP TIME: 10 MINUTES • COOK TIME: 10 MINUTES
LOW-CARB • LOW-FAT/LOW-CHOLESTEROL • LOW-SODIUM

5-INGREDIENT, 30 MINUTES OR LESS, ONE-POT

This dish is well seasoned with onions and a mildly spicy barbeque blend, and then brought together by sweet bell peppers and fresh lime juice. Swap the bell peppers for a poblano pepper for a richer, earthier, and more subtle, spicy flavor. Add these delicious fajitas to a whole wheat soft taco with avocado and shredded lettuce or add them to a lettuce cup instead. Garnish with cilantro for a refreshing finish.

8 ounces chicken breast, cut into 1-inch strips

1 small onion, diced (about ⅓ cup)

1 teaspoon Barbeque Seasoning Rub Blend (page 158)

1 teaspoon avocado oil

2 bell peppers (any color), cut into ½-inch strips

¼ teaspoon freshly ground black pepper

Juice of 1 lime (about 2 tablespoons)

1. In a large freezer bag, combine the chicken, onion, and barbeque seasoning until all the chicken pieces are fully coated. Let the chicken marinate while prepping the other ingredients, or prepare beforehand and let it marinate longer for flavor enhancement.

2. In a medium skillet, heat the oil over medium heat. Add the bell peppers and black pepper and cook for about 5 minutes, until the bell peppers are sizzling and fork-tender.

3. Add the chicken mixture and stir occasionally for another 5 minutes, or until the chicken cooks through. Add the lime juice and serve. Store this dish in an airtight container in the refrigerator for up to 3 days.

MAKE IT EASIER TIP: Marinate the chicken breast, onion, avocado oil, bell peppers, and black pepper in oil and the barbeque seasoning for at least 10 to 15 minutes. Bake in a casserole dish at 400°F for 30 to 35 minutes, until the peppers are charred and the chicken cooks through. Garnish with lime juice.

Per serving: Calories: 202, Total fat: 6g, Saturated fat: 1g, Cholesterol: 80mg, Sodium: 57mg, Potassium: 345mg, Magnesium: 21mg, Carbohydrates: 12g, Sugars: 7g, Fiber: 4g, Protein: 27g, Added sugar: 0g, Vitamin K: 0mcg

One-Skillet Chicken, Green Beans, and Pine Nuts

SERVES 2 • PREP TIME: 5 MINUTES • COOK TIME: 15 MINUTES
LOW-CARB • LOW-FAT/LOW-CHOLESTEROL • LOW-SODIUM

5-INGREDIENT, 30 MINUTES OR LESS, ONE-POT

Lean chicken breast is paired with crisp green beans and toasted pine nuts, then seasoned with garlic and basil in this one-pot meal. Pine nuts' buttery taste comes from their fat content, which is heart-healthy, monounsaturated, anti-inflammatory, and LDL reducing. Be sure to flatten the chicken prior to cooking to reduce cooking time and avoid burning the pine nuts.

2 teaspoons avocado oil

3 garlic cloves, minced

1½ cups green beans, cut into 2-inch pieces

1 tablespoon unsalted raw pine nuts

8 ounces chicken breast, cut into 6 even strips

¼ teaspoon freshly ground black pepper

1 tablespoon finely chopped fresh basil

1. In a medium skillet, heat the oil and garlic over medium heat, until the garlic is fragrant and translucent, 1 to 2 minutes.

2. Add the green beans and pine nuts and cook for about 3 minutes, until the green beans begin to soften and are slightly fork-tender.

3. Add the chicken and season with the pepper and basil. Cook for 3 minutes on one side until ¼ inch of the bottom of the chicken turns white.

4. Flip the chicken, stir the ingredients, and cook for an additional 3 to 5 minutes until the chicken has cooked through. Divide between two serving plates and serve. This dish can also be stored in the refrigerator in an airtight container for up to 3 days, although it is best served warm.

MAKE IT EASIER TIP: Place these ingredients in a casserole dish to cook and forget about it. Bake at 400°F for 25 to 30 minutes, until the green beans are lightly golden and fork-tender and the chicken is lightly browned and cooked through.

Per serving: Calories: 228, Total fat: 10g, Saturated fat: 2g, Cholesterol: 80mg, Sodium: 58mg, Potassium: 211mg, Magnesium: 31mg, Carbohydrates: 8g, Sugars: 3g, Fiber: 3g, Protein: 27g, Added sugar: 0g, Vitamin K: 45mcg

Stuffed Chicken Breast with Spinach and Arugula-Basil Pesto

SERVES 2 • PREP TIME: 10 MINUTES • COOK TIME: 20 MINUTES
LOW-CARB • LOW-FAT/LOW-CHOLESTEROL • LOW-SODIUM

5-INGREDIENT, 30 MINUTES OR LESS, ONE-POT

This chicken breast is moist, juicy, and flavorful. It is stuffed with a fresh arugula pesto sauce and perfectly cooked spinach for a bite that melts in your mouth and keeps you asking for more. I like to pair this dish with the Watermelon Gazpacho (page 64) in the summer or the Cannellini Bean and Swiss Chard Soup (page 67) in the winter. It is also an easy meal to pair with ½ cup of quinoa and Chile-Lime Glazed Brussels Sprouts (page 73).

2 (4-ounce) chicken breasts

1 cup fresh spinach

1 tablespoon Arugula-Basil Pesto (page 161)

2 teaspoons paprika

1. Preheat the oven to 375°F. Line a baking sheet with parchment paper.

2. Pound each chicken breast flat with a meat tenderizer or a rolling pin (covered in plastic wrap) until the breast is even and thin.

3. In a small bowl, combine the spinach and pesto.

4. Place the chicken breasts on the prepared baking sheet and divide the spinach mixture to evenly place half inside the middle of each tender.

5. Fold the chicken breasts in half and rub 1 teaspoon of paprika on the outside of each chicken breast. Cook for 20 minutes until the chicken is cooked through. Serve on a plate with a side dish of your choice. This dish can be stored in an airtight container in the refrigerator for up to 3 days.

SUBSTITUTION TIP: Swap the Arugula-Basil Pesto for the Cashew Cream Dressing (page 164) for a nuttier, cheesier flavor.

Per serving: Calories: 190, Total fat: 9g, Saturated fat: 1g, Cholesterol: 80mg, Sodium: 65mg, Potassium: 174mg, Magnesium: 25mg, Carbohydrates: 3g, Sugars: 1g, Fiber: 2g, Protein: 27g, Added sugar: 0g, Vitamin K: 210mcg

Blueberry, Pistachio, and Parsley Chicken

SERVES 2 • PREP TIME: 5 MINUTES • COOK TIME: 25 MINUTES

LOW-CARB • LOW-FAT/LOW-CHOLESTEROL • LOW-SODIUM

5-INGREDIENT, 30 MINUTES OR LESS, ONE-POT

The smell of this dish cooking will fill your home with delicious flavors. The blueberries paired with the balsamic vinegar create a sweet, caramelized topping that is well balanced by parsley, black pepper, and crunchy pistachios. This dish goes beautifully over a bed of spinach and additional fresh berries—the juices from the chicken will dress the spinach and the fresh berries will add texture to the dish.

½ cup blueberries

2 tablespoons shelled unsalted raw pistachios

¼ cup chopped fresh parsley

2 tablespoons balsamic vinegar

¼ teaspoon freshly ground black pepper

2 (4-ounce) pieces of chicken

1. Preheat the oven to 375°F. Line a baking dish with parchment paper.

2. In a medium mixing bowl, mix the blueberries, pistachios, parsley, vinegar, and pepper until well combined.

3. Put the chicken in the baking dish and pour the blueberry mixture on top. Bake for 20 to 25 minutes, depending on the thickness of the chicken (20 minutes for 1-inch-thick chicken, 25 minutes for 2-inch-thick chicken), until the juices are caramelized and the inside of the chicken has cooked through. Serve on a plate with a side dish of your choice. Store in the refrigerator in an airtight container for up to 3 days.

SUBSTITUTION TIP: To change up the flavor profile, swap the blueberries for strawberries and the pistachios for walnuts.

Per serving: Calories: 212, Total fat: 7g, Saturated fat: 1g, Cholesterol: 80mg, Sodium: 58mg, Potassium: 171mg, Magnesium: 18mg, Carbohydrates: 11g, Sugars: 7g, Fiber: 2g, Protein: 27g, Added sugar: 0g, Vitamin K: 138mcg

Chicken Cacciatore

SERVES 2 • PREP TIME: 5 MINUTES • COOK TIME: 10 MINUTES

LOW-CARB • LOW-FAT/LOW-CHOLESTEROL • LOW-SODIUM

30 MINUTES OR LESS, ONE-POT

Cacciatore means "hunter" in Italian and characterizes a tomato-based stew. This rendition has a bit of a twist—olives and sun-dried tomatoes are added for a brothy, savory, and aromatic pairing. These sweet and savory flavors shine and blend together for a very flavorful dish. Pair this with a refreshing Radish, Cucumber, and Mint Salad (page 48).

2 teaspoons avocado oil

½ cup diced yellow onion

1 cup baby portabella mushrooms, thinly sliced

2 tablespoons low-sodium Kalamata olives, chopped

4 tablespoons low-sodium sun-dried tomatoes, thinly sliced

2 (4-ounce) chicken breasts

½ teaspoon freshly ground black pepper

1 cup no-salt-added tomato sauce

1. In a medium skillet, heat the oil and onions over medium heat for 2 minutes until the onion is translucent.

2. Add the mushrooms, olives, and sun-dried tomatoes. Cook for 1 minute, until the mushrooms are tender.

3. Add the chicken and season with pepper. Cook on one side for 4 minutes until ¼-inch of the bottom of the chicken turns white and the bottom is lightly browned.

4. Flip the chicken, add the tomato sauce, and mix well. Cook for 2 to 3 minutes, until the chicken is cooked through. Portion, plate, and serve. This dish can be stored in an airtight container in the refrigerator for up to 3 days.

FLAVOR TIP: To add more richness and deeper flavor, stir in ½ cup of red wine after step 3. Cook, stirring, for a few minutes, until the wine has reduced by about half. Follow with step 4.

Per serving: Calories: 283, Total fat: 9g, Saturated fat: 1g, Cholesterol: 80mg, Sodium: 208mg, Potassium: 509mg, Magnesium: 24mg, Carbohydrates: 21g, Sugars: 11g, Fiber: 5g, Protein: 30g, Added sugar: 0g, Vitamin K: 11mcg

Zucchini-Chicken Kabobs with Roasted Tomatoes

SERVES 4 • PREP TIME: 10 MINUTES • COOK TIME: 15 MINUTES
LOW-CARB • LOW-FAT/LOW-CHOLESTEROL • LOW-SODIUM

5-INGREDIENT, 30 MINUTES OR LESS, ONE-POT

Growing up, my mom always roasted tomatoes to make a sweet, caramelized sauce to coat kabobs. The tomato juice makes these chicken kabobs moist, and the Mediterranean spice blend makes this a warm, aromatic dish. This dish pairs well with ½ cup of brown rice or Roasted Summer Squash Farro Salad (page 59).

1 pound lean ground chicken or turkey breast

1 cup shredded zucchini

½ cup yellow finely diced onion

1 tablespoon Mediterranean Seasoning Rub Blend (page 159)

1 cup cherry tomatoes

1. Set an oven rack 6 inches from the broiler and preheat the oven to broil. Line a baking sheet with parchment paper.

2. In a medium mixing bowl, mix the chicken, zucchini, onion, and seasoning blend. Let marinate for at least 10 minutes.

3. Scoop 1 heaping tablespoon of the chicken mixture and form the mixture into 1-inch meatballs, making about 8 balls. Add the cherry tomatoes to the parchment paper.

4. Broil for 5 to 7 minutes on one side until lightly golden brown. Flip the rectangles and cook for an additional 4 to 5 minutes until golden brown and juicy. The tomatoes should be blistered. Serve with a whole grain side of your choice. This dish can be stored in an airtight container in the refrigerator for up to 3 days.

FLAVOR TIP: Add ½ teaspoon of sumac to the spice blend or after these are cooked for a tangy, lemony flavor. Sumac is a common spice in Persian culture, and kabobs are often sprinkled with it. You can find this spice at international Middle Eastern specialty stores, and it's worth a trip for this dish!

Per serving: Calories: 169, Total fat: 5g, Saturated fat: 1g, Cholesterol: 90mg, Sodium: 107mg, Potassium: 509mg, Magnesium: 16mg, Carbohydrates: 6g, Sugars: 3g, Fiber: 2g, Protein: 24g, Added sugar: 0g, Vitamin K: 7mcg

Turkey Cauliflower Burgers

SERVES 4 • PREP TIME: 10 MINUTES • COOK TIME: 15 MINUTES

LOW-CARB • LOW-FAT/LOW-CHOLESTEROL • LOW-SODIUM

5-INGREDIENT, 30 MINUTES OR LESS

These juicy burgers are seasoned with a flavor-forward Mediterranean blend and are a hit with my whole family, especially my 2-year-old son, Jacob. I packed these burgers with vitamin C–rich cauliflower and potassium-rich frozen spinach to add a heart-healthy boost and bind the burger. Garnish this dish with sliced red onion, tomato, and fresh spinach, or pair it with Cauliflower Steak with Arugula-Basil Pesto (page 72).

2 cups cauliflower florets (about ½ medium cauliflower head)

1 small yellow onion, quartered

8 ounces frozen spinach, thawed

1 pound lean ground turkey

1½ teaspoons Mediterranean Seasoning Rub Blend (page 159)

1. Set an oven rack 6 inches from the broiler and preheat the oven to broil. Line a baking sheet with parchment paper.

2. In a blender, pulse the cauliflower and onion for 1 to 2 minutes, until they are minced.

3. In a large mixing bowl, combine the spinach, cauliflower and onion mixture, turkey, and the spice blend. Mix well and form into 8 medium patties and place them on the baking sheet.

4. Broil for 10 minutes on one side, flip when lightly golden and juicy, and then broil for 3 minutes on the other side until golden brown. Serve on a whole wheat bun with lettuce and tomato, on top of a salad, or in a collard green wrap. The burgers can be stored in the refrigerator in an airtight container for up to 3 days or frozen for up to 3 months.

SUBSTITUTION TIP: Swap the cauliflower for 1 cup of broccoli florets for a greener and slightly firmer burger. Broccoli has more vitamin K than cauliflower, so be mindful if you are tracking your vitamin K intake.

Per serving (2 burgers): Calories: 206, Total fat: 10g, Saturated fat: 3g, Cholesterol: 84mg, Sodium: 134mg, Potassium: 600mg, Magnesium: 69mg, Carbohydrates: 7g, Sugars: 2g, Fiber: 3g, Protein: 25g, Added sugar: 0g, Vitamin K: 216mcg

Blueberry and Pumpkin Seed Yogurt Bark

PAGE 149

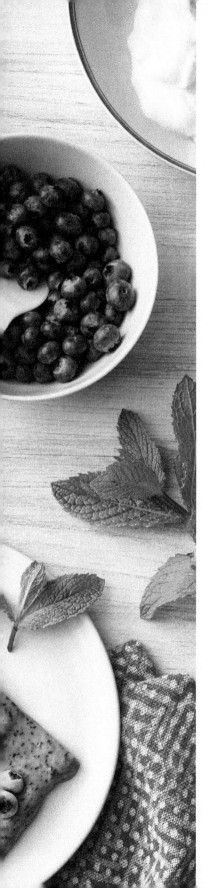

Eight

SWEET TREATS AND SAVORY SNACKS

Pear with Cinnamon-Spiced Walnut Butter

SERVES 4 • PREP TIME: 15 MINUTES • COOK TIME: 25 MINUTES
LOW-SODIUM • VEGAN

5-INGREDIENT, ONE-POT

Toasted walnuts are blended to smooth perfection with sweet cinnamon and woodsy vanilla to make a rich walnut butter perfect for pears. I particularly like this walnut butter with the semi-tart, soft, and juicy Green Anjou variety, though any pear will work. The walnut butter also goes well on top of fluffy Chia Seed, Blueberry, and Yogurt Pancakes (page 36) or the Pineapple-Banana Muffins (page 147).

1 cup raw walnuts

1 teaspoon ground cinnamon

¼ teaspoon pure vanilla extract

4 pears, cored and sliced

1. Preheat the oven to 425°F. Line a baking sheet with parchment paper and spread out the walnuts. Bake for 5 minutes until the walnuts become lightly golden brown.

2. Into the large bowl of a food processor, put the walnuts, cinnamon, and vanilla. Blend for 15 to 18 minutes, until the walnuts turn into a butter-like consistency. It will be clumpy, then will eventually turn into a creamy nut butter consistency. Just be patient and pause to scrape down the sides as needed.

3. Add 1 tablespoon of walnut butter to 1 sliced pear. Store the walnut butter in an airtight container in the refrigerator for up to 1 week.

MAKE IT EASIER TIP: If in a pinch, in a mixing bowl, combine 4 tablespoons of room-temperature unsalted, raw, creamy almond butter with cinnamon and vanilla until well mixed.

Per serving (1 tablespoon): Calories: 297; Total fat: 19g; Saturated fat: 2g; Cholesterol: 0mg; Sodium: 3mg; Potassium: 432mg; Magnesium: 92mg; Carbohydrates: 32g; Sugars: 18g; Fiber: 8g; Protein: 5g; Added sugar: 0g; Vitamin K: 9mcg

Cantaloupe Slices with Blackberry Balsamic Glaze

SERVES 2 • PREP TIME: 15 MINUTES • COOK TIME: 15 MINUTES
LOW-FAT/LOW-CHOLESTEROL • LOW-SODIUM • VEGAN

5-INGREDIENT, 30 MINUTES OR LESS, ONE-POT

A sophisticated and easy-to-make balsamic glaze accompanies a juicy, sweet cantaloupe for a savory and sweet dessert duo. Cantaloupe has one of the highest beta-carotene concentrations found in fruit—hence its beautiful orange color—and is jam-packed with vitamin C, potassium, and folate. When the balsamic vinegar is cooked down, it turns sweet and gains a syrup-like texture. This dish is best served immediately to ensure its sweetness and glaze-like consistency.

1 cup blackberries, mashed

½ cup balsamic vinegar

½ teaspoon pure maple syrup

2 cups cubed cantaloupe

1. In a small pot over medium heat, mix the blackberries, vinegar, and maple syrup well and bring to a boil. Then, turn the heat to low and simmer for 10 to 15 minutes, until the mixture reduces by half and thickens into a glaze.

2. To serve, divide the cantaloupe into two bowls and drizzle the glaze on top. The glaze will thicken and lose its sweetness as it sits, so be sure to serve immediately.

FLAVOR TIP: Add 2 tablespoons of fresh mint or fresh basil to the glaze for a refreshing effect.

Per serving: Calories: 146; Total fat: 1g; Saturated fat: <1g; Cholesterol: 0mg; Sodium: 41mg; Potassium: 619mg; Magnesium: 42mg; Carbohydrates: 32g; Sugars: 27g; Fiber: 5g; Protein: 3g; Added sugar: 1g; Vitamin K: 19mcg

Chocolate Mousse

SERVES 6 • PREP TIME: 5 MINUTES

LOW-CARB • LOW-SODIUM • VEGETARIAN

5-INGREDIENT, 30 MINUTES OR LESS, ONE-POT

A traditional chocolate mousse is high in artery-clogging saturated fat and sugar from the heavy cream, whipped cream, and added sugar. This recipe mimics a mousse's texture and flavor, while protecting your heart—thick, smooth, and chocolaty with subtle hints of vanilla, honey, and cinnamon. I advise you to portion the mixture into small ramekins to keep yourself from eating the whole mixture all at once—it's that good!

1 (3.5-ounce) bar 70-percent dark chocolate

1 (14-ounce) package extra-firm tofu, excess water drained and tofu patted dry

1 teaspoon pure vanilla extract

1 teaspoon honey

1 teaspoon cinnamon

1. In a medium microwave-safe bowl, heat the chocolate bar in the microwave in 30-second increments until the bar has melted, about 2 minutes.

2. In a blender, blend the tofu, vanilla, honey, cinnamon, and melted chocolate until smooth, about 1 minute, scraping down the sides as needed. Serve as is.

3. The mousse can be stored in an airtight container in the refrigerator for up to 3 days. The mixture may thicken slightly as it cools.

SUBSTITUTION TIP: For a looser, less thick but still velvety mousse, substitute the extra-firm tofu for silken tofu. Chill in the refrigerator for 30 to 60 minutes, until the desired consistency is achieved.

Per serving: Calories: 131; Total fat: 18g; Saturated fat: 4g; Cholesterol: 1mg; Sodium: 11mg; Potassium: 292mg; Magnesium: 57mg; Carbohydrates: 9g; Sugars: 5g; Fiber: 2g; Protein: 6g; Added sugar: 1g; Vitamin K: 2mcg

Strawberry-Apple Crumble

SERVES 6 • PREP TIME: 10 MINUTES • COOK TIME: 50 MINUTES

LOW-SODIUM • VEGAN

ONE-POT

Baking this crumble will fill your home with delectable apple and cinnamon scents. The sweet Fuji apples and fresh strawberries cook down so that their sugars caramelize and flavors blend to form a comforting bite. They're then topped with a crisp crumble made of buttery pecans, warm cinnamon, and spicy nutmeg. This dish is a crowd-pleaser and pairs well with a dollop of nonfat Greek yogurt on top. Enjoy it warm or cold.

¼ cup almond meal

¾ cup quick-cooking oats

2 teaspoons pure maple syrup

1 tablespoon avocado oil

1½ teaspoons ground cinnamon, divided

¼ teaspoon ground nutmeg

¼ cup pecan pieces

3 Fuji apples, thinly sliced

2 cups strawberries, quartered

1. Preheat the oven to 400°F.

2. In a medium mixing bowl, combine the almond meal, oats, maple syrup, oil, 1 teaspoon of cinnamon, the nutmeg, and pecan.

3. In a 9-inch round, oven-safe dish, put the apples, strawberries, and the remaining ½ teaspoon of cinnamon and stir until the fruit is well coated.

4. Top the fruit with the crumble mixture and bake for 45 to 50 minutes, until the top is lightly golden, the fruit bubbles, and the apples have softened. Divide into 6 small bowls and serve. The crumble can be stored in the refrigerator in an airtight container for up to 4 days. It will get a bit softer as it sits; warm it up in the oven on broil for 5 minutes to crisp it up again.

FLAVOR TIP: You can use three of the same apples or mix a variety of apples for a slightly different flavor profile. If you want a more tart crumble, add Granny Smith apples. If you want a lightly tart but mostly sweet apple, try Honeycrisp. If you want a crisper apple, try Golden Delicious—but check the dish at around 40 minutes to see if the apples have softened; different apples may take different amounts of time to cook.

Per serving: Calories: 201; Total fat: 9g; Saturated fat: 1g; Cholesterol: 0mg; Sodium: 4mg; Potassium: 279mg; Magnesium: 45mg; Carbohydrates: 29g; Sugars: 16g; Fiber: 5g; Protein: 3g; Added sugar: 1g; Vitamin K: 3mcg

Chocolate Chip and Carrot Cookie

SERVES 8 • PREP TIME: 10 MINUTES • COOK TIME: 20 MINUTES

LOW-CARB • LOW-SODIUM • VEGETARIAN

30 MINUTES OR LESS, ONE-POT

This fluffy, airy dessert is a mix between a chocolate chip cookie and a carrot cake. It has a bittersweet profile from the dark chocolate chips, which is complemented by the earthy carrots and light sweetness of applesauce, maple syrup, and warm cinnamon. I created these cookies for Valentine's Day for my husband and formed them into heart shapes. They were a big hit!

1¼ cups almond meal

½ teaspoon baking powder

¼ cup dark chocolate chips

½ cup shredded carrots

¼ cup unsweetened applesauce

2 teaspoons pure maple syrup

1 whole egg

1 teaspoon cinnamon

1. Preheat the oven to 375°F. Line a baking sheet with parchment paper.

2. In a large mixing bowl, combine the almond meal, baking powder, chocolate chips, carrots, applesauce, maple syrup, egg, and cinnamon until the mixture becomes a thick, doughy consistency.

3. With a tablespoon, scoop out the dough and form the cookies into your desired shape and place on the baking sheet. Bake for 10 to 15 minutes until the cookies puff up, are lightly golden brown, and a fork comes out clean when inserted into a cookie's center. Store in an airtight container in the refrigerator for up to 4 days.

SUBSTITUTION TIP: If you want to create a more savory flavor profile and add a nice crunch to your cookie, swap the dark chocolate chips for raw cacao nibs or crushed cacao beans. They are low in sugar and high in heart-protective nutrients: magnesium, manganese, and copper.

Per serving: Calories: 150; Total fat: 12g; Saturated fat: 2g; Cholesterol: 21mg; Sodium: 61mg; Potassium: 167mg; Magnesium: 52mg; Carbohydrates: 11g; Sugars: 6g; Fiber: 2g; Protein: 5g; Added sugar: 1g; Vitamin K: 1mcg

Pineapple-Banana Muffins

SERVES 8 • PREP TIME: 10 MINUTES • COOK TIME: 20 MINUTES

LOW-FAT/LOW-CHOLESTEROL • LOW-SODIUM • VEGAN

30 MINUTES OR LESS

This pineapple-banana muffin is a hearty, comforting, fluffy, and airy treat. The pineapples add a sweet-tart caramelized note and moisten the muffin, while complementing the fruity banana beautifully. Cinnamon, vanilla extract, and a touch of maple syrup sweeten the dessert and bring all the flavors together in a beautiful union. For a decadent treat, add 1 teaspoon of Cinnamon-Spiced Walnut Butter (see page 142) on top of the warm muffin add ¼ cup of cacao powder, 2 tablespoons of water, and ¼ cup of chocolate chips to the batter.

2 tablespoons ground flaxseed

5 tablespoons water

2 cups oat flour

1 tablespoon cinnamon

1 teaspoon baking powder

1 cup mashed banana (about 3 medium-size ripe bananas)

2 tablespoons pure maple syrup

½ cup crushed pineapple (in 100-percent juice), packed

1 teaspoon pure vanilla extract

¼ cup walnut pieces

1. Preheat the oven to 375°F. In a muffin tin, line 8 muffin cups.

2. In a small mixing bowl, stir the flaxseed and water and let sit for 5 minutes, until the mixture congeals.

3. In a large mixing bowl, combine the flour, cinnamon, and baking powder and mix well.

4. In a medium mixing bowl, stir the flaxseed mixture, bananas, maple syrup, pineapple, and vanilla. Mix well and then slowly pour the wet ingredients into the dry ingredients. Mix in the walnut.

5. Evenly distribute the mixture into the lined muffin tin, filled to the top if possible, and bake for 20 minutes, until the muffin tops are golden brown and a fork inserted into the center comes out clean. Store in an airtight container in the refrigerator for up to 5 days. These are best served warm, so reheat them in the microwave in 15-second increments until the desired temperature is met.

Per serving: Calories: 199; Total fat: 5g; Saturated fat: 1g; Cholesterol: 0mg; Sodium: 64mg; Potassium: 260mg; Magnesium: 57mg; Carbohydrates: 34g; Sugars: 9g; Fiber: 5g; Protein: 6g; Added sugar: 3g; Vitamin K: 2mcg

Peanut Butter and Chocolate Black Bean Brownie

SERVES 6 • PREP TIME: 10 MINUTES • COOK TIME: 15 MINUTES
LOW-CARB • LOW-SODIUM • VEGAN

5-INGREDIENT, 30 MINUTES OR LESS, ONE-POT

Nobody will guess that these brownies are made from black beans; they're likely to impress any chocolate lover. Black beans add a fudgy consistency that resembles that of a feel-good brownie dessert. Fiber-rich black beans are sweetened with potassium-rich dates, melted antioxidant-rich dark chocolate, and copper-rich peanuts. These ingredients come together to form a moist, soft, delicious brownie.

1 (15-ounce) can low-sodium black beans, drained and rinsed

6 small dates, halved

1½ ounces (about half a bar) 70-percent dark chocolate bar, quartered

2 tablespoons quick-cooking oats

2 tablespoons unsalted raw peanut butter

2 tablespoons water

1. Preheat the oven to 350°F.

2. In a medium bowl for a food processor, combine the black beans, dates, chocolate, oats, peanut butter, and water. Blend until very smooth and doughy, 2 to 3 minutes.

3. Pour the batter to an 8-inch square baking pan and spread evenly. Cook for about 15 minutes until the top turns a darker brown, is cracked, and a fork comes out clean when inserted in the middle.

4. Let cool for at least 5 minutes before cutting into 6 squares. Store in an airtight container for up to 3 days on the counter.

FLAVOR TIP: To add a nice crunch to the brownies, stir 2 tablespoons of chopped walnuts or peanuts into the batter before you cook it.

Per serving: Calories: 160; Total fat: 6g; Saturated fat: 2g; Cholesterol: <1mg; Sodium: 3mg; Potassium: 299mg; Magnesium: 53mg; Carbohydrates: 22g; Sugars: 7g; Fiber: 7g; Protein: 6g; Added sugar: 0g; Vitamin K: 2mcg

Blueberry and Pumpkin Seed Yogurt Bark

SERVES 6 • PREP TIME: 5 MINUTES, PLUS 2 TO 4 HOURS TO CHILL

LOW-CARB • LOW-FAT/LOW-CHOLESTEROL • LOW-SODIUM • VEGETARIAN

5-INGREDIENT, ONE-POT

If you love froyo, ice cream, or frozen treats, this dessert is for you! Plain yogurt is blended with refreshing mint, sweet blueberries, and a hint of honey—all topped with crunchy pumpkin seeds and whole blueberries that add a nice texture. This bark can also be an easy breakfast alternative that balances high-quality protein, dietary fiber, and heart-healthy fats! Eat this delicious snack in a bowl to catch the yogurt bark liquid goodness as it melts. Add a drizzle of dark chocolate for extra decadence.

2 cups nonfat plain yogurt

1¼ cups blueberries, divided

1 tablespoon coarsely chopped fresh mint

1 teaspoon honey

¼ cup raw unsalted pumpkin seeds

1. Line a baking sheet with parchment paper, making sure the edges are covered.

2. In a medium bowl for a food processor, combine the yogurt, 1 cup of blueberries, the mint, and honey. Blend until smooth, about 2 minutes.

3. Using a rubber spatula, evenly spread the yogurt mixture over the parchment paper.

4. Evenly add the remaining ¼ cup of blueberries and pumpkin seeds on top of the yogurt mixture.

5. Freeze for 2 to 4 hours, until the bark is fully frozen. The best way to check is to poke the middle of the pan with a fork to see if it has hardened. Once fully frozen, the edges should easily lift as well.

6. Break the bark up into 12 pieces and freeze in an airtight container or freezer-safe zip-top bag for up to 1 month.

Per serving: Calories: 95; Total fat: 3g; Saturated fat: 1g; Cholesterol: 2mg; Sodium: 64mg; Potassium: 273mg; Magnesium: 45mg; Carbohydrates: 13g; Sugars: 10g; Fiber: 1g; Protein: 6g; Added sugar: 1g; Vitamin K: 6mcg

Raspberry-Lime Sorbet

SERVES 2 • PREP TIME: 5 MINUTES, PLUS 2 TO 4 HOURS TO CHILL

LOW-FAT/LOW-CHOLESTEROL • LOW-SODIUM • VEGETARIAN

5-INGREDIENT, ONE-POT

Berries are my dessert favorite—not just for their delicious fruity flavor and varying levels of tartness but for their heart-healthy, antioxidant-rich, anti-inflammatory, and anticoagulant profile. This is a refreshing, tart raspberry iced dessert with a citrus-y note and a sweet touch of honey. It acts as a beautiful palate cleanser, especially after a heavy meal.

2 cups frozen raspberries

2 teaspoons honey

1 teaspoon lime juice

½ cup warm water

1. In a blender, blend the raspberries, honey, lime juice, and water on high for 2 to 3 minutes until well combined.

2. Place the mixture in a freezer-safe cup or in a ice-pop mold. Freeze 2 to 4 hours until firm. Store in the freezer in an airtight container for up to 1 month.

SUBSTITUTION TIP: For a sweeter treat, swap the lime juice for Meyer lemon juice and the honey for maple syrup.

Per serving: Calories: 162; Total fat: 2g; Saturated fat: <1g; Cholesterol: 0mg; Sodium: 10mg; Potassium: 464mg; Magnesium: 58mg; Carbohydrates: 37g; Sugars: 22g; Fiber: 11g; Protein: 3g; Added sugar: 6g; Vitamin K: 11mcg

Whole Wheat Seed Crackers

SERVES 4 • PREP TIME: 10 MINUTES • COOK TIME: 20 MINUTES

LOW-FAT/LOW-CHOLESTEROL • LOW-SODIUM • VEGAN

5-INGREDIENT, 30 MINUTES OR LESS, ONE-POT

These crispy crackers are flavored with a savory blend of garlic and za'atar, a Middle Eastern aromatic spice composed of toasted sesame seeds, earthy thyme and oregano, and citrus-y lemon peel. The crackers' crunch makes them a perfect dipping vehicle for Artichoke-Basil Hummus (page 154), Edamame-Guacamole Dip (page 155), or the Tofu-Chive Cream Cheese (page 170). You can also cut the cracker dough into long crisp breads and use it as a substitute for bread.

1 cup whole wheat flour

2 tablespoons ground flaxseed

2 tablespoons hemp seeds

1 tablespoon za'atar
(see Substitution Tip, page 83)

2 teaspoons garlic powder

½ cup water

1. Preheat the oven to 400°F. Line a baking sheet with parchment paper.

2. In a large mixing bowl, mix the flour, flaxseed, hemp seeds, za'atar, garlic powder, and water until it is dough-like and slightly sticky.

3. Using a rolling pin or a floured wine bottle, spread the dough to a thickness of about one-tenth of an inch. Cut the dough into bite-size crackers (about 1-by-1-inch) and separate them to allow crispy edges to form on each cracker.

4. Bake for 20 minutes until lightly browned and the edges are crispy. Store in an airtight container for up to 1 week.

SUBSTITUTION TIP: Swap out 1 tablespoon of hemp seeds for 1 tablespoon of psyllium husk powder for a boost of pure soluble fiber. Psyllium husk does not add any flavor but may make the cracker crisper.

Per serving (10 crackers): Calories: 163; Total fat: 5g; Saturated fat: 1g; Cholesterol: 0mg; Sodium: 36mg; Potassium: 188mg; Magnesium: 77mg; Carbohydrates: 25g; Sugars: <1g; Fiber: 5g; Protein: 7g; Added sugar: 0g; Vitamin K: 1mcg

Roasted Cannellini Bean "Chips"

SERVES 6 • PREP TIME: 5 MINUTES • COOK TIME: 20 MINUTES
LOW-CARB • LOW-FAT/LOW-CHOLESTEROL • LOW-SODIUM • VEGAN

5-INGREDIENT, 30 MINUTES OR LESS, ONE-POT

These crunchy cannellini beans are a perfect substitution for popcorn. They are crispy on the outside and soft on the inside. These nutty beans have a smoky taste with a hint of cinnamon and a subtle, refreshing lemon aftertaste. Batch-cook them and keep them around to snack on, or add as a crunchy topping to salads such as the Mediterranean Cucumber, Tomato, and Kalamata Olive Salad (page 58). These are also a great addition to any crudité platter or for guests to munch on instead of salted nuts.

2 cups low-sodium cannellini beans, drained and rinsed

2 tablespoons avocado oil

1 tablespoon lemon juice

½ teaspoon smoked paprika

½ teaspoon ground cumin

½ teaspoon ground cinnamon

1. Preheat the oven to 425°F. Line a baking sheet with parchment paper.

2. In a medium mixing bowl, combine the beans, oil, lemon juice, paprika, cumin, and cinnamon.

3. Spread the beans onto the prepared baking sheet in one even layer, and roast for 20 minutes until the beans become crispy and flaky.

SUBSTITUTION TIP: Replace the cinnamon with dried thyme for a more savory citrus flavor.

Per serving: Calories: 108; Total fat: 5g; Saturated fat: 0.5g; Cholesterol: 0mg; Sodium: 27mg; Potassium: 266mg; Magnesium: 62mg; Carbohydrates: 12g; Sugars: 1g; Fiber: 3g; Protein: 4g; Added sugar: 0g; Vitamin K: 4mcg

Cheesy Kale Chips

SERVES 4 • PREP TIME: 10 MINUTES • COOK TIME: 15 MINUTES

LOW-CARB • LOW-SODIUM • VEGAN

5-INGREDIENT, 30 MINUTES OR LESS, ONE-POT

These kale chips are crunchy and cheesy, and one of the best things I've ever eaten. Lacinato kale cooks down into a flat, crispy chip and is deliciously flavored by tahini and B-vitamin-rich nutritional yeast that forms a paste that acts like nacho cheese on top of the kale chips. I should warn you: These chips go fast and you may want to make a double batch because they won't last. When adding the paste to the kale chips, be sure to evenly distribute it into a thin layer so that the chips stay crispy and the "cheese" mixture melts down completely.

4 tablespoons unsalted tahini

4 heaping tablespoons nutritional yeast

½ teaspoon garlic powder

½ cup water

1 large bunch of kale, cut into 2-inch chunks (about 5 tightly packed cups)

1. Preheat the oven to 400°F. Line a baking sheet with parchment paper.

2. In a large mixing bowl, combine the tahini, nutritional yeast, garlic powder, and water. The consistency should be runny enough to spread evenly over the kale.

3. Add the kale to the tahini mixture, thinly coating each kale piece, avoiding any clumpy chunks of sauce. Transfer the dipped kale to the prepared baking sheet and spread so that the pieces don't touch.

4. Bake for 10 to 15 minutes, until the edges become slightly browned and the kale turns into a crispy chip. Serve alongside your favorite main dish or enjoy as a crunchy snack. Store in a large container for up to 3 days; the crispiness starts to fade in 24 hours.

SUBSTITUTION TIP: Swap the tahini for unsalted sunflower seed butter for a more mild, roasted taste.

Per serving: Calories: 130; Total fat: 9g; Saturated fat: 1g; Cholesterol: 0mg; Sodium: 34mg; Potassium: 318mg; Magnesium: 33mg; Carbohydrates: 8g; Sugars: 1g; Fiber: 5g; Protein: 8g; Added sugar: 0g; Vitamin K: 370mcg

Artichoke-Basil Hummus

SERVES 8 • PREP TIME: 15 MINUTES

LOW-CARB • LOW-SODIUM • VEGAN

30 MINUTES OR LESS, ONE-POT

An artichoke dip meets a citrus-y tahini-based hummus in this dish. The delicious, mildly nutty undertone of the artichokes blends with fresh, peppery basil, and a creamy blend of chickpeas, tahini, and bright lemon juice. This dish is easily paired with the crunchy crudité of your choice, homemade Whole Wheat Seed Crackers (page 151), or as part of the protein source of Hummus and Greens Pasta (page 95). You can also thin it out and use as a sauce or dressing with a salad.

1 (15-ounce) can low-sodium chickpeas, drained and rinsed

¼ cup unsalted tahini

2 garlic cloves

3 tablespoons lemon juice

3 tablespoons extra-virgin olive oil

1 cup frozen artichoke pieces, defrosted

3 tablespoons chopped fresh basil

4 tablespoons water

Freshly ground black pepper

In a blender, blend the chickpeas, tahini, garlic, lemon juice, olive oil, artichoke, basil, water, and pepper until smooth.

MAKE IT EASIER TIP: Frozen artichoke pieces are low-sodium; canned artichokes are not. Thaw frozen artichokes overnight and use 1 tablespoon of dried basil for fresh basil and 1 teaspoon of garlic powder to make meal prep time even shorter.

Per serving (¼ cup): Calories: 242; Total fat: 16g; Saturated fat: 2g; Cholesterol: 0mg; Sodium: 51mg; Potassium: 258mg; Magnesium: 28mg; Carbohydrates: 20g; Sugars: 3g; Fiber: 7g; Protein: 7g; Added sugar: 0g; Vitamin K: 53mcg

Edamame-Guacamole Dip

SERVES 6 • PREP TIME: 10 MINUTES

LOW-CARB • LOW-SODIUM • VEGAN

5-INGREDIENT, 30 MINUTES OR LESS, ONE-POT

This guacamole has the perfect texture—creamy from the ripe, rich, and buttery avocado, chunky from the pulsed edamame, and crunchy from the red bell peppers. I enjoy this dip paired with Whole Wheat Seed Crackers (page 151) and my favorite crudité trio—fresh cauliflower, carrots, and asparagus. This edamame-guacamole dip can also give a nice flavor boost to the Tofu-Chive Cream Cheese Sandwich (page 100) instead of avocados, or to the Salmon Tacos with Cabbage Slaw (page 106).

2 medium avocados, ripe

½ cup frozen cooked
  edamame, thawed

½ medium red bell pepper,
  diced (½ cup)

2 tablespoons lime juice

¼ cup packed cilantro,
  leaves only

½ teaspoon freshly ground
  black pepper

In a medium bowl for a food processor, pulse the avocados, edamame, bell pepper, lime juice, cilantro, and black pepper until the desired consistency is achieved, 10 to 15 seconds.

FLAVOR TIP: To add some heat, blend in ½ jalapeño pepper with 1 teaspoon of low-sodium hot sauce.

Per serving (¼ cup): Calories: 146; Total fat: 11g; Saturated fat: 2g; Cholesterol: 0mg; Sodium: 11mg; Potassium: 402mg; Magnesium: 23mg; Carbohydrates: 10g; Sugars: 1g; Fiber: 6g; Protein: 4g; Added sugar: 0g; Vitamin K: 6mcg

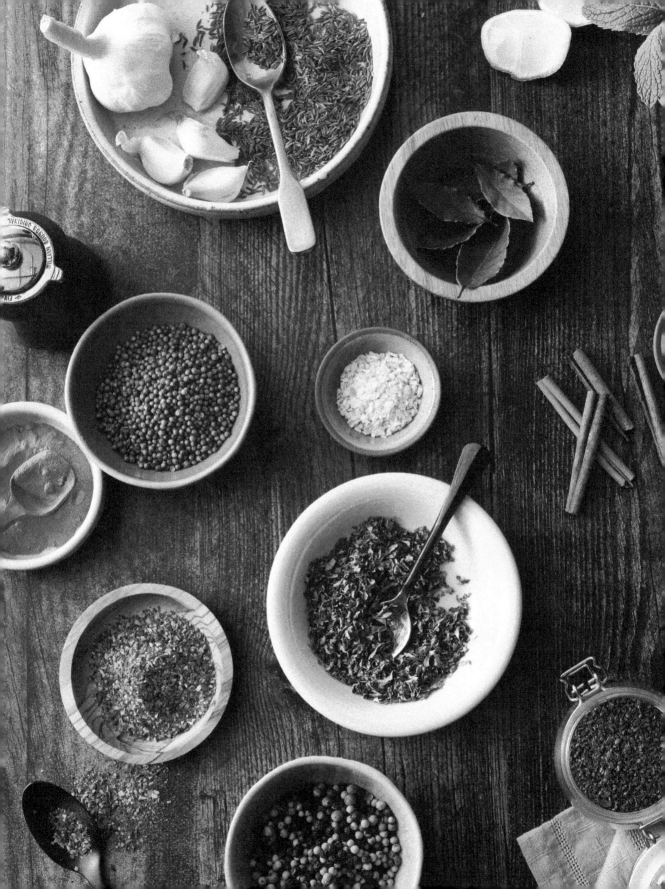

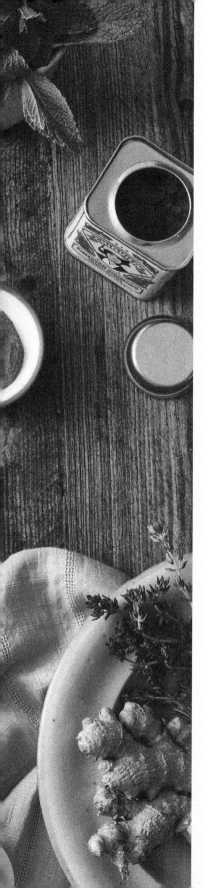

Nine

SEASONINGS, SAUCES, AND STAPLES

Barbeque Seasoning Rub Blend

YIELDS 1 TABLESPOON AND ½ TEASPOON • PREP TIME: 5 MINUTES
LOW-CARB • LOW-FAT/LOW-CHOLESTEROL • LOW-SODIUM • VEGAN

5-INGREDIENT, 30 MINUTES OR LESS, ONE-POT

Aromatic and smoky paprika blends with nutty cumin, spicy cayenne pepper, savory garlic, and sweet onion powder to mimic a delicious barbeque seasoning with medium heat. If you like more heat, increase the cayenne pepper to 1 teaspoon, and if you desire less, reduce it to ⅛ teaspoon or omit it completely.

2 teaspoons smoked paprika

1 teaspoon ground cumin

½ teaspoon cayenne pepper

½ teaspoon garlic powder

½ teaspoon onion powder

In an empty spice container, mix the paprika, cumin, cayenne pepper, garlic powder, and onion powder until well combined.

FLAVOR TIP: Add ½ teaspoon of mustard powder to the barbeque seasoning for mild heat and an added tanginess.

Per serving (¼ teaspoon): Calories: 1.5; Total fat: 0g; Saturated fat: 0g; Cholesterol: 0mg; Sodium: 0.5mg; Potassium: 6mg; Magnesium: 1mg; Carbohydrates: 0g; Sugars: 0g; Fiber: 0g; Protein: 0g; Added sugar: 0g; Vitamin K: 0mcg

Mediterranean Seasoning Rub Blend

YIELDS 2 TABLESPOONS • PREP TIME: 5 MINUTES

LOW-CARB • LOW-FAT/LOW-CHOLESTEROL • LOW-SODIUM • VEGAN

5-INGREDIENT, 30 MINUTES OR LESS, ONE-POT

Dried garlic powder meets spicy black pepper, earthy turmeric, smoky rich paprika, and cumin in a blend of spices that adds a warm flavor profile to any dish. This spice blend is versatile and can be used to flavor any vegetable or protein from lentils and black beans to fish and lean chicken breast.

2 teaspoons garlic powder

1½ teaspoon freshly ground black pepper

1 teaspoon ground turmeric

½ teaspoon smoked paprika

½ teaspoon ground cumin

In an empty spice container, mix the garlic powder, pepper, turmeric, paprika, and cumin until well combined.

SUBSTITUTION TIP: If the cumin is a bit too nutty for your taste, swap it for ground caraway seeds. Caraway seeds have a milder flavor, but impart the same note.

Per serving (¼ teaspoon): Calories: 2; Total fat: 0g; Saturated fat: 0g; Cholesterol: 0mg; Sodium: 0mg; Potassium: 8mg; Magnesium: 1mg; Carbohydrates: <1g; Sugars: 0g; Fiber: 0g; Protein: 0g; Added sugar: 0g; Vitamin K: 0mcg

Chile-Lime Glaze

YIELDS 2 TABLESPOONS • PREP TIME: 5 MINUTES

LOW-CARB • LOW-FAT/LOW-CHOLESTEROL • LOW-SODIUM • VEGAN

5-INGREDIENT, 30 MINUTES OR LESS, ONE-POT

This light dressing has a subtle spicy hint that is balanced with a touch of pure maple syrup and a citrus-y lime note. This dish enhances the flavor of many dishes, from the Tempeh Taco Salad with Chile-Lime Glaze (page 60) to the Chile-Lime Tempeh Tacos with Green Apple Slaw (page 98), to the Cilantro-Lime Chicken (page 128). If you aren't heating the oil, swap the avocado oil for olive oil to achieve a richer flavor profile.

1 tablespoon avocado oil

⅛ teaspoon red pepper flakes

2 tablespoons lime juice
(about 1 lime)

1 teaspoon pure maple syrup

In a medium mixing bowl, combine the oil, red pepper flakes, lime juice, and maple syrup. Store in an airtight container in the refrigerator for up to 1 week.

SUBSTITUTION TIP: To increase the heat, add another ¼ teaspoon of red pepper flakes. To decrease it, substitute the red pepper flakes for chile powder. While chile powder still contains ground hot pepper, it is tempered by other spices such as garlic and onion powder.

Per serving (1 tablespoon): Calories: 48; Total fat: 5g; Saturated fat: 1g; Cholesterol: 0mg; Sodium: 1mg; Potassium: 16mg; Magnesium: 1mg; Carbohydrates: 2g; Sugars: 2g; Fiber: 0g; Protein: 0g; Added sugar: 1g; Vitamin K: 0mcg

Arugula-Basil Pesto

YIELDS 4½ TABLESPOONS • PREP TIME: 10 MINUTES

LOW-CARB • LOW-SODIUM • VEGAN

5-INGREDIENT, 30 MINUTES OR LESS, ONE-POT

I have never found a low-sodium store-bought pesto. This light, refreshing version was my solution to that and is made with peppery arugula, sweet basil, and buttery walnuts. You can easily thin the consistency of the pesto for a flavorful salad dressing or thicken by using less water for a paste-like sauce. It pairs well with Cauliflower Steak with Arugula-Basil Pesto (page 72) and Salmon Tacos with Cabbage Slaw (page 106). This pesto is an easy-to-make kitchen staple that will definitely be a crowd-pleaser!

1½ cups arugula, stems trimmed

½ cup basil, stems trimmed

¼ cup unsalted raw walnuts, coarsely chopped

2 garlic cloves

2 tablespoons extra-virgin olive oil

¼ teaspoon freshly ground black pepper

¼ teaspoon ground cumin

3 tablespoons water

In a medium bowl for a food processor combine the arugula, basil, walnuts, garlic, olive oil, pepper, cumin, and water for 1 to 2 minutes, until the desired consistency is achieved. Store in the refrigerator in an airtight container for up to 5 days.

SUBSTITUTION TIP: Swap out the arugula for spinach for a lighter, greener taste.

Per serving (1 tablespoon): Calories: 101; Total fat: 10g; Saturated fat: 1g; Cholesterol: 0mg; Sodium: 3mg; Potassium: 76mg; Magnesium: 17mg; Carbohydrates: 2g; Sugars: <1g; Fiber: 1g; Protein: 1g; Added sugar: 0g; Vitamin K: 20mcg

Chimichurri Sauce

YIELDS ⅜ CUP • PREP TIME: 10 MINUTES

LOW-CARB • LOW-SODIUM • VEGAN

5-INGREDIENT, 30 MINUTES OR LESS, ONE-POT

Chimichurri is an uncooked herb sauce originating in Argentina. It is typically paired with meat, but deliciously coats lean protein, whole grains, vegetables, or salads for a simple flavor enhancement. This rendition stays true to its flavor as a light, refreshing, and tangy sauce used in the Pan-Seared Salmon with Chimichurri Sauce (page 110) and the Broiled Tofu, Pepper, and Onions with Chimichurri Sauce (page 93).

¼ cup extra-virgin olive oil

1 tablespoon red wine vinegar

1 garlic clove, minced

½ cup chopped fresh parsley

1 teaspoon dried oregano

⅛ teaspoon red pepper flakes

In a medium mixing bowl, combine the olive oil, vinegar, garlic, parsley, oregano, and red pepper flakes and mix well. Store in an airtight container in the refrigerator for up to 1 week.

SUBSTITUTION TIP: While green chimichurri is more commonly recognized in the United States, you can make this into a red chimichurri sauce similar to red salsa. Substitute ¼ cup of the parsley with ¼ cup of red bell peppers and substitute the oregano with smoked paprika.

Per serving (1 tablespoon): Calories: 83; Total fat: 9g; Saturated fat: 1g; Cholesterol: 0mg; Sodium: 3mg; Potassium: 33mg; Magnesium: 3mg; Carbohydrates: 1g; Sugars: <1g; Fiber: <1g; Protein: <1g; Added sugar: 0g; Vitamin K: 88mcg

Cilantro-Mint Sauce

YIELDS ½ CUP • PREP TIME: 10 MINUTES

LOW-CARB • LOW-FAT/LOW-CHOLESTEROL • LOW-SODIUM • VEGETARIAN

30 MINUTES OR LESS, ONE-POT

This refreshing, citrus-y, and zesty sauce is a bright and cooling addition to any dish. Creamy yogurt is blended with mint and cilantro and added to lemon juice, ginger, and honey for a balanced and delicious combination. This dish can be easily used to garnish hot dishes after cooking, or to help flavor any salad, side, or main dish. Cilantro-mint sauce is a key ingredient in the Collard Green Halibut Wraps with Cilantro-Mint Sauce (page 113) and Roasted Eggplant and Chickpeas with Cilantro-Mint Sauce (page 86).

½ cup nonfat plain Greek yogurt

2 tablespoons lemon juice

1 medium bunch of cilantro, stemmed (about 3 cups)

1 cup mint leaves

1-inch piece ginger, grated

1 teaspoon honey

1 to 2 tablespoons water (optional)

1. In a medium bowl for a food processor, blend the yogurt, lemon juice, cilantro, mint, ginger, and honey for 1 to 2 minutes, until combined and the desired texture is achieved.

2. If making a sauce, add 1 to 2 tablespoons of water. If you prefer as a relish, don't add any water. Store in the refrigerator in an airtight container for up to 5 days.

MAKE IT EASIER TIP: Purchase pre-grated ginger, usually found in the frozen aisle, and add 1 frozen cube into this dish. You can also prep ginger in bulk by peeling the whole bulb, breaking it into 1-inch pieces, and placing it in a food processor. Once you've grated the whole bulb, pack it into ice cube trays and freeze. Once frozen, remove the cubes and put in a freezer-safe bag for future use.

Per serving (2 tablespoons): Calories: 32; Total fat: <1g; Saturated fat: <1g; Cholesterol: 2mg; Sodium: 21mg; Potassium: 154mg; Magnesium: 12mg; Carbohydrates: 5g; Sugars: 3g; Fiber: 1g; Protein: 4g; Added sugar: 1g; Vitamin K: 37mcg

Cashew Cream Dressing

YIELDS ½ CUP • PREP TIME: 5 MINUTES

LOW-CARB • LOW-SODIUM • VEGAN

5-INGREDIENT, 30 MINUTES OR LESS, ONE-POT

An extra-creamy vegan take on a classic cheese sauce, this recipe brings a welcome addition to any dish when you want a home-cooked, comfort-food feel. Creamy cashews rich in copper, manganese, and magnesium blend well with thick oat milk and are flavored with cheesy, savory nutritional yeast and an earthy cumin undertone. This dish is essential for a delicious Creamed Spinach (page 66), Tofu with Mushroom Cream Sauce (page 94), and Fish Florentine (page 118).

1 cup raw cashews

⅓ cup plus 1 tablespoon unsweetened oat milk

2 tablespoons nutritional yeast

1 garlic clove, smashed

¼ teaspoon freshly ground black pepper

¼ teaspoon ground cumin

Blend the cashews, oat milk, nutritional yeast, garlic, pepper, and cumin in a high-speed blender for about 2 minutes, until smooth. Store in an airtight container in the refrigerator for up to 1 week. The sauce may thicken in the refrigerator; if it does, add 1 tablespoon of warm water and mix well.

FLAVOR TIP: Roast the garlic if you want an added boost of flavor. To roast one garlic clove, add 1 teaspoon of avocado oil to a small skillet, heat for about 1 minute on medium heat, and add the smashed garlic clove and stir until lightly browned, 3 to 4 minutes.

Per serving (2 tablespoons): Calories: 206; Total fat: 15g; Saturated fat: 2.5g; Cholesterol: 0mg; Sodium: 16mg; Potassium: 335mg; Magnesium: 101mg; Carbohydrates: 12.5g; Sugars: 2g; Fiber: 2.5g; Protein: 8.5g; Added sugar: 0g; Vitamin K: 6.5mcg

Tahini-Garlic Dressing

YIELDS ¼ CUP • PREP TIME: 5 MINUTES

LOW-CARB • LOW-SODIUM • VEGAN

5-INGREDIENT, 30 MINUTES OR LESS, ONE-POT

Ground sesame seeds are the base of this delicious dressing. With an added touch of olive oil, a splash of citrus, a note of peppery, well-textured stone-ground mustard, and savory garlic, these ingredients come together to make a versatile dressing and sauce that complements most dishes. It is a staple I highly recommend batch-cooking.

2 tablespoons unsalted tahini

½ tablespoon extra-virgin olive oil

Juice of 1 lemon

1 teaspoon stone-ground mustard seed

2 garlic cloves, minced

¼ teaspoon freshly ground black pepper

1 tablespoon cold water, plus more as needed

In a medium mixing bowl combine the tahini, olive oil, lemon juice, mustard, garlic, pepper, and water and mix well. For a thinner dressing, add more water until the desired consistency is achieved. Store in an airtight container for up to 5 days in the refrigerator.

FLAVOR TIP: Add 1 teaspoon of maple syrup or honey to add a bit of sweetness to balance out the tangy, savory notes.

Per serving (2 tablespoons): Calories: 135; Total fat: 12g; Saturated fat: 2g; Cholesterol: 0mg; Sodium: 61mg; Potassium: 118mg; Magnesium: 18mg; Carbohydrates: 7g; Sugars: 1g; Fiber: 2g; Protein: 3g; Added sugar: 0g; Vitamin K: 2mcg

Ginger-Sesame Dressing

YIELDS ¼ CUP • PREP TIME: 5 MINUTES

LOW-CARB • LOW-FAT/LOW-CHOLESTEROL • LOW-SODIUM • VEGAN

5-INGREDIENT, 30 MINUTES OR LESS, ONE-POT

Typical sesame dressing is high in sodium from the soy sauce (even the low-salt varieties are high in salt). This dressing is well balanced, low in sodium, and adds flair to just about any dish. Toasted sesame oil is aromatically pleasing and adds a meaty flavor that is balanced by tangy rice vinegar, zesty ginger, and crunchy sesame seeds.

2 tablespoons toasted sesame oil

2 teaspoons rice vinegar

2 teaspoons fresh grated ginger

2 teaspoons unsalted
sesame seeds

In a small bowl, mix the sesame oil, rice vinegar, ginger, and sesame seeds until well combined. Store in the refrigerator in an airtight container for up to 1 week.

FLAVOR TIP: For added heat, add ½ teaspoon of hot sauce and 1 teaspoon of lime juice to balance it out.

Per serving (1 tablespoon): Calories: 66; Total fat: 7g; Saturated fat: 1g; Cholesterol: 0mg; Sodium: 1mg; Potassium: 14mg; Magnesium: 2mg; Carbohydrates: 1g; Sugars: <1g; Fiber: <1g; Protein: <1g; Added sugar: 0g; Vitamin K: 1mcg

Tzatziki Dip

YIELDS 2 CUPS • PREP TIME: 10 MINUTES

LOW-CARB • LOW-FAT/LOW-CHOLESTEROL • LOW-SODIUM • VEGETARIAN

5-INGREDIENT, 30 MINUTES OR LESS, ONE-POT

Tzatziki is my ultimate favorite dipping sauce. I frequently prepare it for my husband and kids to have a delicious, well-balanced dip available, and use the yogurt container to reduce cleanup. This tzatziki sauce is creamy, fresh, and cooling. The grated cucumber adds a refreshing note alongside the citrus-y lemon juice, lemon zest, and grassy fresh dill.

1 medium cucumber, grated

Juice and zest of 1 large lemon
(3 tablespoons lemon juice and
1 teaspoon lemon zest)

1 tablespoon fresh dill, minced

1 teaspoon freshly ground
black pepper

2 cups 0, 1 or 2 percent plain
Greek Yogurt

1. Place the grated cucumber in a paper towel and squeeze to drain out the water.

2. In a medium mixing bowl or yogurt container, combine the cucumber, lemon juice, lemon zest, dill, pepper, and yogurt and stir until the ingredients come together. Store in the refrigerator for up to 5 days.

FLAVOR TIP: For the flavors to marinate and deeply develop, tightly cover and refrigerate for 4 hours or overnight. Mix well when ready to eat.

Per serving (½ cup): Calories: 74; Total fat: <1g; Saturated fat: <1g; Cholesterol: 6mg; Sodium: 44mg; Potassium: 244mg; Magnesium: 20mg; Carbohydrates: 6g; Sugars: 4g; Fiber: <1g; Protein: 12g; Added sugar: 0g; Vitamin K: 10mcg

Tartar Sauce

YIELDS 1 CUP • PREP TIME: 10 MINUTES

LOW-CARB • LOW-FAT/LOW-CHOLESTEROL • LOW-SODIUM • VEGETARIAN

5-INGREDIENT, 30 MINUTES OR LESS, ONE-POT

Traditional tartar sauce contains heavily processed ingredients, preservatives, and fat. This tartar sauce is creamy from the yogurt, slightly salty from the dill pickles, and fresh and savory from the parsley and onions. Add this to Fish and Chips with Homemade Tartar Sauce (page 120) and Buffalo Tofu and Cauliflower Bites (page 85) and Salmon Burgers with Homemade Yogurt Mustard Sauce (page 108) or carrots and celery for a well-balanced snack.

1 cup nonfat plain Greek yogurt

¼ cup chopped dill pickles

2 tablespoons finely chopped fresh parsley

¼ teaspoon freshly ground black pepper

1 teaspoon lemon juice

1 teaspoon grated onion

In a medium mixing bowl, stir the yogurt, pickles, parsley, pepper, lemon juice, and onion until well combined.

SUBSTITUTION TIP: For a tangier tartar sauce, add 1 teaspoon of Dijon mustard.

Per serving (¼ cup): Calories: 39; Total fat: <1g; Saturated fat: <1g; Cholesterol: 3mg; Sodium: 96mg; Potassium: 112mg; Magnesium: 9mg; Carbohydrates: 3g; Sugars: 2g; Fiber: <1g; Protein: 6g; Added sugar: 0g; Vitamin K: 33mcg

Barbeque Sauce

YIELDS 1½ CUPS • PREP TIME: 5 MINUTES • COOK TIME: 10 MINUTES

LOW-CARB • LOW-FAT/LOW-CHOLESTEROL • LOW-SODIUM • VEGAN

30 MINUTES OR LESS, ONE-POT

Traditional barbeque sauce is high in salt and sugar; this recipe is not! This easy-to-make, low-sodium, low-sugar barbeque sauce has a complex smoky but sweet flavor with subtle heat. You can easily increase the heat by adding more cayenne pepper or decrease the heat by omitting it completely. Using minimal yet bold ingredients, this barbeque sauce is a flavor-forward, multi-use kitchen staple everyone will enjoy.

2 tablespoons whole wheat flour

¼ cup water

1 tablespoon and ½ teaspoon Barbeque Seasoning Rub Blend (page 158)

2 cups no-salt-added tomato sauce

1 tablespoon pure maple syrup

1 tablespoon Dijon mustard

2 garlic cloves, minced

1. In a small mixing bowl, combine the whole wheat flour and water. Mix until there are no clumps.

2. In a medium pot, combine the flour-water mixture with the seasoning blend, tomato sauce, maple syrup, mustard, and garlic and simmer over medium heat for 5 to 10 minutes, until the sauce thickens. Store in the refrigerator in an airtight container for up to a week.

FLAVOR TIP: To make this tangier, add in ¼ cup of apple cider vinegar.

Per serving (2 tablespoons): Calories: 29; Total fat: <1g; Saturated fat: 0g; Cholesterol: 0mg; Sodium: 38mg; Potassium: 24mg; Magnesium: 4mg; Carbohydrates: 4g; Sugars: 3g; Fiber: 1g; Protein: 1g; Added sugar: 1g; Vitamin K: 1mcg

Tofu-Chive Cream Cheese

YIELDS 2 CUPS • PREP TIME: 10 MINUTES

LOW-CARB • LOW-FAT/LOW-CHOLESTEROL • LOW-SODIUM • VEGAN

5-INGREDIENT, 30 MINUTES OR LESS, ONE-POT

Traditional cream cheese is very high in saturated fat and nutritionally unbalanced, leaving you hungry shortly after. This recipe blends tofu, a lean high-quality protein, with chives, nutritional yeast, olive oil, and apple cider vinegar to create a flavor-forward, savory spread. It is easily used as a dish's main protein or as a delicious dipping sauce for a snack.

1 (14-ounce) package extra-firm tofu

¼ cup chopped fresh chives

¼ cup extra-virgin olive oil

2 teaspoons nutritional yeast

1 tablespoon apple cider vinegar

¼ teaspoon freshly ground black pepper

1. Press the tofu to remove excess moisture by gently squeezing it between two sheets of paper towel.

2. In a blender, blend the tofu, chives, olive oil, nutritional yeast, vinegar, and pepper for 1 to 3 minutes, until well combined and a creamy consistency has formed. Store in the refrigerator in an airtight container for up to 5 days.

FLAVOR TIP: Add 1 tablespoon of fresh dill for a lemon-y, refreshing twist.

Per serving (2 tablespoons): Calories: 59; Total fat: 5g; Saturated fat: 1g; Cholesterol: 0mg; Sodium: 2mg; Potassium: 41mg; Magnesium: 1mg; Carbohydrates: 1g; Sugars: 0g; Fiber: <1g; Protein: 3g; Added sugar: 0g; Vitamin K: 2mcg

Chia Berry Jam

YIELDS 1 CUP • PREP TIME: 5 MINUTES, PLUS OVERNIGHT TO CHILL

LOW-CARB • LOW-FAT/LOW-CHOLESTEROL • LOW-SODIUM • VEGAN

5-INGREDIENT, 30 MINUTES OR LESS, ONE-POT

Mildly nutty chia seeds bind together with a variety of sweet, tart, acidic frozen berries to create a perfect jam. This dish can be used to top the Chia Seed, Blueberry, and Yogurt Pancakes (page 36) or whole wheat toast. To make it sweeter, mix in a teaspoon of pure maple syrup, honey, or date syrup.

1½ cups frozen mixed berries

¼ cup chia seeds

½ cup water

1. In a medium glass storage container, put the mixed berries, chia seeds, and water. Close the storage container tightly with a secure lid and shake thoroughly. Chill the mixture overnight in the refrigerator.

2. In the morning, using a fork, mix and mash the chia berry mixture to the desired consistency. Store in an airtight container in the refrigerator for up to 5 days.

SUBSTITUTION TIP: To add a sweet, tangy taste, substitute the water for ½ cup of juiced orange with ¼ teaspoon of orange zest.

Per serving (2 tablespoons): Calories: 43; Total fat: 2g; Saturated fat: 0g; Cholesterol: 0mg; Sodium: 3mg; Potassium: 0mg; Magnesium: 0mg; Carbohydrates: 6g; Sugars: 2g; Fiber: 3g; Protein: 1g; Added sugar: 0g; Vitamin K: 1mcg

Homemade Vegetable Broth

YIELDS ABOUT 6 CUPS • PREP TIME: 10 MINUTES • COOK TIME: 45 MINUTES

LOW-CARB • LOW-FAT/LOW-CHOLESTEROL • LOW-SODIUM • VEGAN

5-INGREDIENT, ONE-POT

Traditional vegetable and chicken broths are high in sodium. This flavorful and aromatic vegetable stock uses five simple, fresh ingredients to deliver a lot of flavor for any recipe that needs vegetable broth. The mushroom imparts a delicious, subtle umami note and the parsley brings balance to the entire stock. Since you are getting rid of the vegetables in the end, you can leave the skins on and chop the vegetables coarsely just to expose their surface area. This soup is a great staple to freeze and use as needed.

1 tablespoon avocado oil

1 large onion, coarsely chopped

2 large carrots, coarsely chopped

4 celery stalks with leaves, coarsely chopped

1 (8-ounce) package cremini mushrooms, halved

1 medium bunch parsley, coarsely chopped

½ teaspoon freshly ground black pepper

8 cups warm water

1. In a 5-quart pot, heat the oil over medium heat. Add the onion, carrots, and celery and sauté for 5 minutes until fragrant.

2. Add the mushrooms, parsley, pepper, and warm water to the soup and stir to combine well.

3. Cover and bring to a light boil. When bubbles begin to form, lower the heat and simmer for 40 minutes. Strain the stock. Store in the refrigerator for up to 7 days or in the freezer for up to 3 months.

FLAVOR TIP: Save your roots as you cook throughout the week—carrot tops, beet tops, onion skins—and freeze them in a freezer-safe zip-top bag. When you are ready to make a stock, add it to the mix for a delicious, complex flavor boost.

Per serving: Calories: 40; Total fat: 2g; Saturated fat: <1g; Cholesterol: 0mg; Sodium: 26mg; Potassium: 232mg; Magnesium: 11mg; Carbohydrates: 4g; Sugars: 2g; Fiber: 1g; Protein: 1g; Added sugar: 0g; Vitamin K: 240mcg

Turkey Cauliflower Burgers

PAGE 139

Measurement Conversions

	US STANDARD	US STANDARD (OUNCES)	METRIC (APPROXIMATE)
VOLUME EQUIVALENTS (LIQUID)	2 TABLESPOONS	1 FL. OZ.	30 ML
	¼ CUP	2 FL. OZ.	60 ML
	½ CUP	4 FL. OZ.	120 ML
	1 CUP	8 FL. OZ.	240 ML
	1½ CUPS	12 FL. OZ.	355 ML
	2 CUPS OR 1 PINT	16 FL. OZ.	475 ML
	4 CUPS OR 1 QUART	32 FL. OZ.	1 L
	1 GALLON	128 FL. OZ.	4 L
VOLUME EQUIVALENTS (DRY)	⅛ TEASPOON		0.5 ML
	¼ TEASPOON		1 ML
	½ TEASPOON		2 ML
	¾ TEASPOON		4 ML
	1 TEASPOON		5 ML
	1 TABLESPOON		15 ML
	¼ CUP		59 ML
	⅓ CUP		79 ML
	½ CUP		118 ML
	⅔ CUP		156 ML
	¾ CUP		177 ML
	1 CUP		235 ML
	2 CUPS OR 1 PINT		475 ML
	3 CUPS		700 ML
	4 CUPS OR 1 QUART		1 L
	½ GALLON		2 L
	1 GALLON		4 L
WEIGHT EQUIVALENTS	½ OUNCE		15 G
	1 OUNCE		30 G
	2 OUNCES		60 G
	4 OUNCES		115 G
	8 OUNCES		225 G
	12 OUNCES		340 G
	16 OUNCES OR 1 POUND		455 G

	FAHRENHEIT (F)	CELSIUS (C) (APPROXIMATE)
OVEN TEMPERATURES	250°F	120°C
	300°F	150°C
	325°F	180°C
	375°F	190°C
	400°F	200°C
	425°F	220°C
	450°F	230°C

References

Meticulous care and effort was put into researching this book. As such, the references list is extensive. You can find a complete list of references at callistomediabooks.com/thetrulyeasyhearthealthycookbook

Index

Acknowledgments

This book could not have been possible without my family—my husband, Barak, thank you for your support, encouragement, and companionship. Life would not be the same without you by my side. To my mom and dad, I cannot thank you enough for all your love and support and for instilling in me the importance of good food, happiness, and family. To my children, thank you for energizing my life in so many ways—you are my everything. To my mom- and dad-in-law, thank you for your support in this journey. To my siblings, Kaila, Esti, Daniela, Adam, and Arik, thank you for making family what it is meant to be. To Nadine Ghantous, my rockstar intern, thank you for your talented assistance on this project. To the Castillo team, especially Britt Bogan, thank you for all you have done to make this book possible and for cheering me on throughout. To my clients and those reading this book, thank you for trusting me with your health—it is my honor to serve you.

About the Author

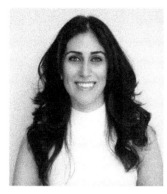

Michelle Routhenstein is a registered dietitian nutritionist, certified diabetes educator, and preventive cardiology dietitian who specializes in heart disease management and prevention. She has a master of science degree in clinical nutrition and completed her nutrition training residency at New York University. She has over 10 years of experience counseling individuals and families on chronic disease prevention and management through personalized, science-based nutrition and lifestyle medicine. She has a thriving nutrition counseling and consulting private practice, in which she sees clients in her New York City office and virtually.

Printed in the USA
CPSIA information can be obtained
at www.ICGtesting.com
CBHW041510220324
5545CB00006B/13